An Illustrated Guide to
Bone Marrow Diagnosis

An Illustrated Guide to
Bone Marrow Diagnosis

Kevin Gatter

BM, DPhil. MRCPath
University Department of Cellular Science
John Radcliffe Hospital, Oxford

David Brown

BSc, MD, MRCPath
Department of Histopathology
Whittington Hospital, London

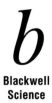

Blackwell
Science

© 1997 by
Blackwell Science Ltd
Editorial Offices:
Osney Mead, Oxford OX2 0EL
25 John Street, London WC1N 2BL
23 Ainslie Place, Edinburgh EH3 6AJ
350 Main Street, Malden
   MA 02148 5018, USA
54 University Street, Carlton
   Victoria 3053, Australia

Other Editorial Offices:
Blackwell Wissenschafts-Verlag GmbH
Kurfürstendamm 57
10707 Berlin, Germany

Blackwell Science KK
MG Kodenmacho Building
7–10 Kodenmacho Nihombashi
Chuo-ku, Tokyo 104, Japan

First published 1997

Set at the Medical Informatics Unit
Department of Cellular Science
University of Oxford
Printed and bound in Italy by
Rotolito Lombarda SpA, Milan

The Blackwell Science logo is a
trade mark of Blackwell Science Ltd,
registered at the United Kingdom
Trade Marks Registry

DISTRIBUTORS

Marston Book Services Ltd
PO Box 269
Abingdon, Oxon OX14 4YN
(*Orders*: Tel: 01235 465500
           Fax: 01235 465555)

USA
Blackwell Science, Inc.
Commerce Place
350 Main Street
Malden, MA 02148 5018
(*Orders*: Tel: 800 759 6102
                 617 388 8250
           Fax: 617 388 8255)

Canada
Copp Clark Professional
200 Adelaide St West, 3rd Floor
Toronto, Ontario M5H 1W7
(*Orders*: Tel: 416 597-1616
                 800 815-9417
           Fax: 416 597-1617)

Australia
Blackwell Science Pty Ltd
54 University Street
Carlton, Victoria 3053
(*Orders*: Tel: 3 9347 0300
           Fax: 3 9347 5001)

A catalogue record for this title
is available from the British Library

ISBN 0-632-04234-6

Contents

Preface

It has been said that the best way to travel is hopefully. Perhaps this is also the best way to write a textbook though I doubt that many authors begin in that way. We set out to write this book on bone marrow pathology because we thought we could write the sort of text that we would want to use ourselves. An inordinate amount of time later and suitably humbled we doubt that we ever want to see this manuscript again. Nevertheless it still approximates to the goal we were seeking. A short text oriented at diagnosis and comprehensively accompanied by usable illustrations. Our aim was to enable a busy pathologist to find on one open page the essential description and illustration of most common bone marrow diseases seen in trephines. We hope we have been successful but welcome comments and criticisms from readers. Who knows we might even produce another edition!

Acknowledgments

It is almost impossible to know where to begin when paying tributes and compliments to one's tutors and colleagues. Many indeed may not want the dubious honour of such recognition. It is impossible to learn anything about bone marrow without the help and tolerance of haematologists so we thank all the many colleagues we have worked with in Oxford over the years. We are both indebted to many histopathologists who tried to teach us the critical examination of tissue slides but all of whom recoiled in horror at looking at trephines. So we are substantially self taught and can only blame ourselves. Three individuals who have stimulated us in different ways often unknowingly need a special mention. They are Michael Dunnill, David Mason and Peter Isaacson. Our thanks to them and to all the others.

The text and image manipulation has all been performed in house in the Department of Cellular Science. This is still a relatively new technology for us and we would not have made any progress without our excellent medical informatics unit run by Kingsley Micklem. We owe a great debt of gratitude to Felicity Williams and Ellie Parker who performed all of the technical work on this project.

K.C.Gatter and D.C. Brown

Introduction

Introduction

During the late 1950s, McFarland and Dameshek introduced an acceptable means of obtaining bone marrow core biopsies.[1] Then it became possible for the histopathologist to diagnose a wide range of haematopathological disorders including the leukaemias, lymphoproliferative and myeloproliferative disease, myelodysplasia, metastases and reactive disorders.

Most biopsies are taken from the posterior superior iliac spine. Ideally in an adult the core of tissue should be at least 1 cm in length. An aspirate is usually taken from the same site before the biopsy is removed. The haematologist will usually make about 10 smear preparations from the marrow particles that have been aspirated and either discard or send the remainder for histology. We find it useful to have both of these types of specimen since there are occasions when only an aspirate is available, in which case it is then important to have built up experience examining aspirate preparations for which trephines have been available for comparison.

The trephine biopsy has a number of advantages over the aspirate specimen. The most important is to enable examination of the topographical distribution of the cellular constituents of the marrow, their relationships to the bony trabeculae and an assessment of marrow cellularity. Furthermore in diseases which produce fibrosis, e.g. Hodgkin's disease, an aspirate often fails to produce an adequate diagnostic sample ('a dry tap').

Close liaison with haematologists is important since it makes the reporting of trephine biopsies easier and ensures that misdiagnoses are kept to a minimum.

There has been debate involving the embedding medium for bone marrow biopsies. There are essentially two schools of thought, those who believe that the biopsies should be embedded in plastic and those who believe paraffin embedding with decalcification to be superior. The reason for this divergence is related to the nature of the biopsy itself which consists of both hard tissue (i.e. bone) and soft tissue (i.e. marrow and fat). In order to cut intact sections one can either make the biopsy material uniformly soft (by decalcification) or uniformly hard (by resin embedding). Unfortunately decalcification inevitably produces some tissue distortion and plastic embedding limits the range of immunohistochemical studies. The debate over which is superior continues with vociferous advocates on either side.[2–6] The advantages and disadvantages of each approach are shown in Table 1.1.

We believe that, with a little extra care, it is possible to provide sections, from paraffin-embedded trephines, which meet the practical requirements of the diagnostic haematologist.[7]

Just as there has been division amongst some pathologists regarding the best embedding medium so too has there been debate over which is the most appropriate general stain. This inevitably involves an element of personal preference. The well-established place of the H&E stain in general diagnostic pathology has assured it of much support amongst pathologists as the primary stain in bone marrow histology. We believe that a good Giemsa stain provides more information than its H&E counterpart, e.g. in identifying cell lineage, the detection of fibrosis, the estimation of iron stores. A good Giemsa stain requires fastidious technical preparation (see chapter 14). The results are worth the initial perseverance on both the part of the technical staff and the pathologist who has to become familiarized with it. When indicated we include a reticulin stain in our bone marrow set.

Reasons for performing bone marrow biopsies

The majority of bone marrow biopsies are performed for the following reasons.[8]

1 Dry tap. The commonest diagnoses are:
  - fibrosis (Hodgkin's, metastatic cancer, primary myelofibrosis);
  - hairy cell leukaemia;
  - extreme hypercellularity ('packed marrow') such as may be seen in cases of leukaemia and lymphoma.

2 Assessment of cellularity:
  - extent of infiltration by leukaemia, lymphoma and myeloma;
  - amount of residual marrow;
  - assessment of marrow post chemotherapy and after engraftment;

Table 1.1 Comparison of the relative advantages and disadvantages of paraffin and plastic embedding of bone marrow trephine biopsies.

	Paraffin embedding	**Resin / plastic embedding**
Advantages	1 Widespread antigen preservation allows immunohisto-chemical studies. 2 Pathologists are familiar with sections cut from paraffin embedded material.	1 Superb cytological detail available from the very thin sections obtained by this technique.
Disadvantages	1 Loss of some histochemical reactivity within the granules of the granulocyte and mast cell series, e.g. Leder stain. This loss is directly proportional to the strength of the acid used in decalcification. 2 Some inevitable tissue distortion is produced by decalcification.	1 Loss of some immunoreactivity. 2 A separate technique is required solely for bone marrow biopsies. 3 Pathologists are unfamiliar with resin embedded sections and their associated artefacts, e.g. the basophilic hue indicative of erythroid histogenesis is lost in resin embedded sections.

Tables 1.2–1.5 A scheme for assessing the bone marrow trephine with some common pathological conditions as examples.

Table 1.2

Assessment of cellularity	
Hypocellular	Aplastic anaemia
	Hairy cell leukaemia
	Acute myeloid leukaemia
Normocellular	Be aware of subtle infiltrates such as myeloma
Hypercellular	
Homogeneous	Non-Hodgkin's lymphoma
	Acute leukaemias
Heterogeneous	Reactive
	Myeloproliferative syndromes
	Myelodysplasias
	Metastatic cancer

Table 1.3

Topography (distribution) of cellular elements

Are all cell types present?
Are any particular cells present in abnormal numbers?
  e.g. increased granulocytes in CGL
  Prominent mast cells in Waldenström's macroglobulinaemia
Normal cellular distribution
  Granulocytes
    Paratrabecular, peri-arterial
  Erythroid
    Intertrabecular
  Megakaryocytes
    Intertrabecular and peri-sinusoidal
Common abnormal patterns
  Myelodysplasia / myeloproliferation
    Paratrabecular erythroid and megakaryocytic colonies
    Megakaryocytic clustering
  Non-Hodgkin's lymphoma
    Follicle centre cell has a paratrabecular pattern
    CLL is usually diffuse or nodular

Tables 1.2–1.5 continued from page 2

Table 1.4

Assessment of cell morphology

Atypia
Abnormal megakaryocytes in myeloproliferation
and myelodysplasia
Maturation abnormalities
Maturation arrest, e.g. drug induced
Asynchronous maturation in myelodysplasia
Abnormal maturation, e.g. megaloblastic anaemia
Imbalance of maturation, e.g. left/right shifted

Table 1.5

Assessment of accessory structures

Vessels
Vasculitis
Amyloid deposition
Sinusoids
Distended in myeloproliferative disorders
Bone
Osteoporosis
Osteomalacia
Paget's
Stroma
Iron deposition
Amyloid
Gelatinous transformation
Granulomas
Fibrosis
Metastatic carcinoma
Gaucher's disease
Organisms
Tuberculosis
Atypical mycobacteria
Leishmaniasis
Histoplasma
Cryptococcus

- investigation of cytopenias.
3 Identification of focal disease:
- metastatic cancer, lymphomas, granulomas.
4 Lymphoma staging.
5 Assessment of HIV infection.

How to examine a trephine section

It is important to have an organized approach to the examination of bone marrow sections in order not to miss diagnostic features. One possible scheme is based on an assessment of cellularity, topography, morphology and accessory structures as illustrated in Tables 1.2–1.5 with a selection of some common pathological conditions.

References

1 McFarland W, Dameshek W. Biopsy of bone marrow with the Vim-Silverman needle. *JAMA* 1958; **166**: 1464–1466.
2 Nand NM. Misunderstandings about methyl methacrylate. *J Clin Pathol* 1993; **46**: 285.
3 Jack AS, Roberts BE, Scott CS. Processing of trephine biopsy specimens. *J Clin Pathol* 1993; **46**: 285.
4 Schmid C, Isaacson PG. Bone marrow trephine biopsy in lympho-proliferative disease. *J Clin Pathol* 1992; **45**: 475–50.
5 Schmid C, Isaacson PG. In reply to correspondence. *J Clin Pathol* 1993; **46**: 285–286.
6 Krenacs T, Krenacs L, Bagdi E. Diagnostic immunocytochemistry in Araldite-embedded bone marrow biopsies. *Cellular Pathol* 1996; **1**: 83–88.
7 Gatter KC, Heryet A, Brown DC, Mason DY. Is it necessary to embed bone marrow biopsies in plastic for haematological diagnosis? *Histopathology* 1987; **11**: 1–7.
8 De Wolf-Peeters C. Bone marrow trephine interpretation; diagnostic utility and pitfalls. Invited review. *Histopathology* 1991; **18**: 489–493.

The normal bone marrow

Chapter 2

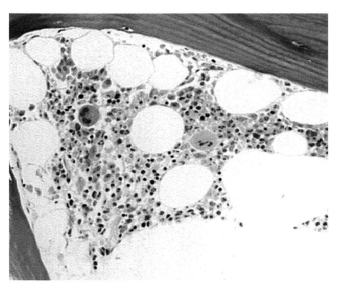

Fig 2.1 Lamellar bone showing parallel lines of ossification. Giemsa.

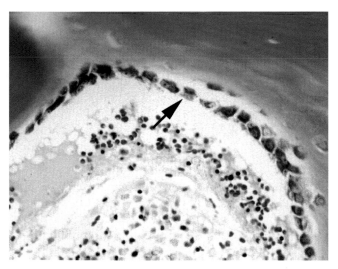

Fig 2.2 Osteoblasts (arrow) along the endosteal surface. Giemsa.

Introduction

The bone marrow is not a random mixture of different blood-forming cells but is a highly organized and specialized tissue. The identification of individual cells is less precise in trephines than smear preparations due to the greater cytological detail present in the latter. Consequently a proportion of the marrow cell population will only be identifiable by the 'company it keeps' or by special staining procedures, notably immunocytochemistry, e.g. stem cells cannot be identified morphologically.[1] Confidence in examining a trephine biopsy is derived from a familiarity with the normal marrow appearances and an understanding of how these alter throughout life.

Site of haematopoiesis

In the normal adult, haematopoiesis is largely restricted to the axial skeleton, i.e. skull, sternum, vertebrae, ribs, pelvis and the proximal regions of the long bones. The marrow in these sites is described as red because of the presence of erythroid elements and in the non-haematopoietic sites as yellow because of the large amount of fat present. Site and cellularity vary with age (Table 2.1).

Components of the normal bone marrow trephine

BONE
STROMA vessels, reticulin, fibroblasts, fat, iron.
HAEMATOPOIETIC TISSUE granulocytic, erythroid,
    megakaryocytic.
OTHER CELLS lymphoid, plasma cells, mast cells.

Bone

The trabeculae consist of lamellar bone (Fig. 2.1). Osteoblasts are present along the endosteal surface (Fig. 2.2). These may superficially resemble plasma cells because of the eccentrically placed nucleus and the presence of a cytoplasmic hof (para-nuclear area of lighter staining cytoplasm). Osteoblasts lack the characteristic 'clock face' nuclear chromatin pattern of plasma cells and the hof of the osteoblast does not abut directly onto the nucleus, but is separated by a narrow rim of darker staining cytoplasm.

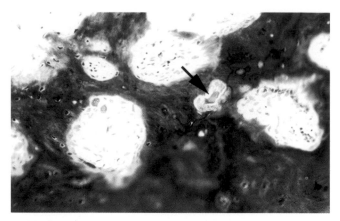

Fig 2.3 Osteoclasts (arrow) housed in Howship's lacuna. Giemsa.

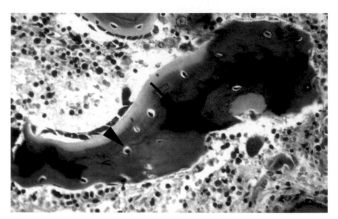

Fig 2.4 Cartilage (arrow) undergoing ossification. Osteocytes (arrowheads) are present within the lacunae. Giemsa.

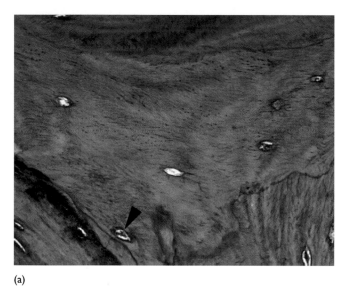

(a)

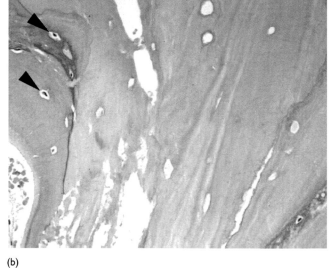

(b)

Fig 2.5 (a) and (b) Necrotic bone. Note the absence of osteocytes in the lacunae. There is a small focus of viable bone where osteocytes are present (arrowheads).

Table 2.1 Bone marrow cellularity.

Age	Site	Cellularity (haemopoietic cells / fat)
Neonate	All bones, liver, spleen	100/0
Child	Most bones	70/30
Adult	Axial skeleton	50/50
Old age	Axial skeleton	30/70

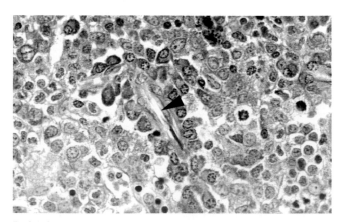

Fig 2.6 Small capillary (arrowhead) surrounded by a thin layer of mature plasma cells. Giemsa.

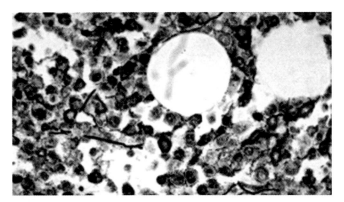

(a) Grade 1. Focal fine reticulin. Normal. Gomori.

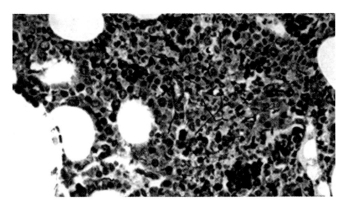

(b) Grade 2. Diffuse fine reticulin. Normal. Gomori.

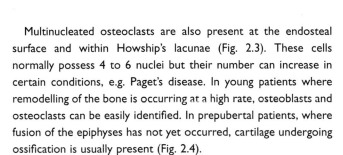

(c) Grade 3. Diffuse fine reticulin, plus focal coarse reticulin. Abnormal. H&E.

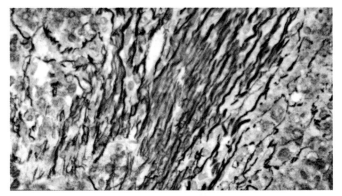

(d) Grade 4. Diffuse coarse reticulin including collagen, i.e. fibrosis. Abnormal. H&E.

Fig 2.7 Semiquantitative grading system of marrow reticulin content.

Multinucleated osteoclasts are also present at the endosteal surface and within Howship's lacunae (Fig. 2.3). These cells normally possess 4 to 6 nuclei but their number can increase in certain conditions, e.g. Paget's disease. In young patients where remodelling of the bone is occurring at a high rate, osteoblasts and osteoclasts can be easily identified. In prepubertal patients, where fusion of the epiphyses has not yet occurred, cartilage undergoing ossification is usually present (Fig. 2.4).

Osteocytes are easily identified within their lacunae (Fig. 2.4). They have densely stained irregular nuclei and because of retraction artefact do not completely fill the lacunae. In necrotic or non-viable bone the osteocytes die and disappear (Fig. 2.5). In elderly patients with osteoporosis the trabeculae are thinned, i.e. generally less than the diameter of a fat cell.

Stroma

VESSELS

Thin-walled venous sinusoids are present throughout the marrow. In the normal marrow they are inconspicuous since they are usually collapsed. This is in contrast to those seen in the myeloprolifer-

ative syndromes where they may be dilated and prominent. They act as the efferent pathway for the mature haematopoietic elements on their way into the general circulation. Mature megakaryocytes are often seen close to or abutting onto the thin walls of these sinusoids, into which they discharge their platelets (Fig. 2.20). Small arteries may also be seen and identified by their relatively thick muscle walls. Granulopoiesis may be seen in proximity to them. Capillaries are easily seen and may be surrounded by a single layer of mature plasma cells, particularly in reactive conditions (Fig. 2.6).

RETICULIN AND FIBROBLASTS

The blood-forming areas of the normal adult marrow have little reticulin and no fibrosis (i.e. fibrosis is regarded as an increase in the number of single reticulin fibres or bundles of fibres to form collagen). The reticulin is produced by inconspicuous elongated fibroblasts and exists as a fine network throughout most of the marrow although it may be condensed and more prominent around arterial vessels. The Gomori silver stain for reticulin readily displays this fine reticulin network, which can be graded semiquantitatively when abnormal (Fig. 2.7).

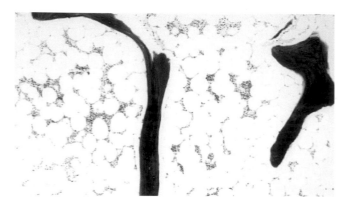

Fig 2.8 Marrow from elderly patient showing increased fat. Giemsa.

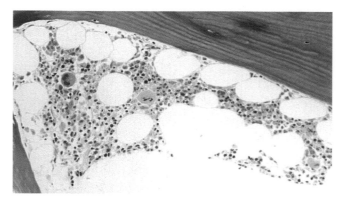

Fig 2.9 Single layer of fat cells separating marrow from the endosteal surface 'first fat space'. Giemsa.

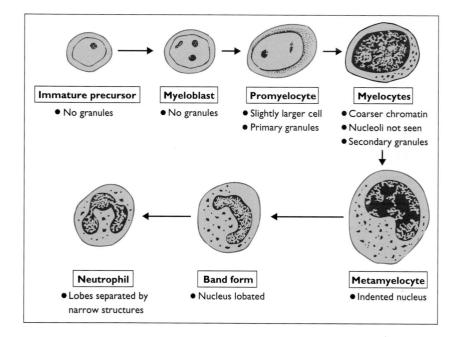

Immature precursor
- No granules

Myeloblast
- No granules

Promyelocyte
- Slightly larger cell
- Primary granules

Myelocytes
- Coarser chromatin
- Nucleoli not seen
- Secondary granules

Neutrophil
- Lobes separated by narrow structures

Band form
- Nucleus lobated

Metamyelocyte
- Indented nucleus

Fig 2.10 Schematic illustration of granulocytic cell differentiation.

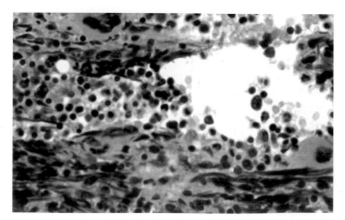

Fig 2.11 Crush artefact mimicking fibrosis. H&E.

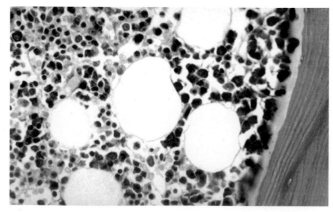

Fig 2.12 Paratrabecular arrangement of granulocytic series immunostained for elastase. APAAP.

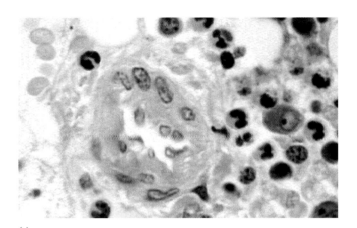
(a)

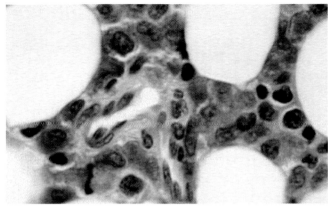
(b)

Fig 2.13 Arteriole with adjacent granulopoiesis. (a) Giemsa. (b) Immunoperoxidase for elastase.

Points to note
- Increased fine and coarse reticulin is present around thick-walled blood vessels.
- Aspirated fragments of marrow tend to contain less reticulin than trephine biopsies. This is because those areas in a marrow with the least reticulin are the most easily aspirated.
- Crush artefact with smearing and elongation of cell nuclei produces a histological picture which may mimic fibrosis (Fig. 2.11). Silver staining is required for differentiation.

FAT

The amount of fat within red marrow increases with age, and consequently the amount of haemopoeitic tissue decreases (Fig. 2.8). In a section of trephine from a normal adult, the fat occupies approximately 50% of the marrow space. The subcortical region of the iliac crest has a greater percentage of fat than deeper regions and hence biopsies containing tissue from the subcortical region should not be misdiagnosed as hypocellular or aplastic. Similarly, there is considerable variation in cellularity throughout a trephine biopsy, a feature which emphasizes the need for an adequately-sized biopsy (>1 cm) that will permit an accurate assessment of the marrow's cellularity. In the normal marrow the cellular elements are separated from the endosteal surface by a single layer of fat cells often referred to as the 'first fat space' (Fig. 2.9). Fat atrophy may occur in hypothyroidism.

IRON

Perls' Prussian blue, which stains haemosiderin, will allow a semi-quantitative assessment of the amount of iron in marrow macrophages. Decalcification causes some loss of iron, so that when indicated, iron stains should be performed on both the aspirate and the trephine biopsy. The Giemsa stain also identifies haemosiderin, producing an olive green coloration of the iron granules.

Haematopoietic tissue

THE GRANULOCYTIC SERIES (Fig. 2.10)

Immature forms of the granulocytic series are arranged along the endosteal surface of the trabeculae with maturation occurring towards the central intertrabecular region (Fig. 2.12). A similar arrangement can also be seen around small arteries within the marrow (Fig. 2.13). Eosinophil precursors can be identified and distinguished from neutrophil precursors by their coarser granules which tend to be refractile and a darker red. Immunohistochemistry can be useful in identifying these cells.

The normal adult marrow has a granulocyte-to-erythroid ratio of approximately 2:1, as assessed by tissue section. In the first few weeks after birth, infants have a reversed ratio with up to 70% of the cells being of the erythroid series, mainly proerythroblasts and normoblasts.

The normal mature neutrophil has up to five nuclear lobes. In tissue sections fewer lobes are seen than in smear preparations since the latter allow whole, intact cells to be visualized. In tissue sections, if more than three lobes can be identified, the neutrophil should be considered hypersegmented. The number of these forms is increased in megaloblastic anaemia.

In marrows with increased numbers of neutrophils, such as in systemic infections or as a reaction to some malignancies, e.g. Hodgkin's disease, the granulocyte series is described as right-shifted. Alternatively an increase in immature forms, for example in an early regenerating marrow or severe infection, is described as left-shifted. A left-shifted granulocytic series is often seen in neonates where promyelocytes and myeloblasts are more obvious than in adult marrow.

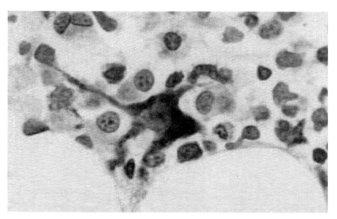

Fig 2.14 Schematic illustration of erythroid differentiation.

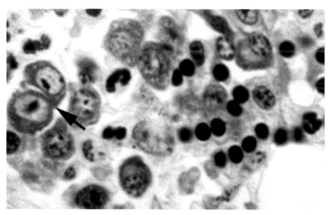

Fig 2.15 Small erythroid island with central macrophage immunostained for CD68. Immunoperoxidase.

Fig 2.16 Erythroid colony showing distinct blueness of erythroblasts (arrow). Giemsa.

A paradox may occur where a patient has a raised white cell count in the peripheral blood but the marrow appears normal. This may be due to administration of steroids which cause demargination of polymorphs from vessel walls into the blood stream.

THE ERYTHROID SERIES (Fig. 2.14)
Erythroid elements are organized into small groups present within the central regions of the marrow and extending up to the first fat space. Within these erythroid islands, all of the elements of this series can be identified, from the early pronormoblast (proerythroblast) through to the normoblast (late erythroblast). Associated with many erythroid islands is a macrophage, usually located centrally and often containing free, stainable iron (Fig. 2.15).

The Giemsa stain imparts a characteristic blueness (Fig. 2.16) to the blast forms of the erythroid series, a feature which is of use in distinguishing them from other immature cell types. This can be helpful in situations such as a marrow regenerating after chemotherapy when the possibility of residual leukaemia is being considered. Paraffin-embedding, but not plastic-embedding, produces an artefactual halo around normoblasts, which is useful in distinguishing them from small lymphocytes (Fig. 2.17).

The normal marrow of a neonate may contain multiple groups of erythroid cells which should not be misinterpreted histologically as metastatic disease (Fig. 2.18).

Erythroid hyperplasia is not uncommon (Table 2.2). Confusion may arise because, in this setting, the erythroid series may show some megaloblastic change. Furthermore, the large numbers of normoblasts present may create a monotonous histological picture superficially similar to CLL. Immunohistochemistry can be particularly valuable in identifying cells of the erythroid series.

THE MEGAKARYOCYTIC SERIES (Fig. 2.19)
Mature megakaryocytes and their precursors are found uniformly distributed throughout the central region of the marrow, particularly in association with thin-walled venous sinuses (Fig. 2.20). Mature megakaryocytes do not usually occur in groups or lie in contact with each other. The presence of more than a few megakaryocytes close to bone trabeculae is abnormal. The mature forms are easily identified on tissue sections since they are the largest cells within the normal marrow. Less mature forms, e.g. megakaryoblasts, are less easily identified using conventional stains but are readily recognized immunohistochemically.

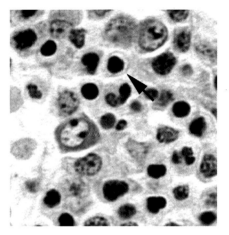

Fig 2.17 Normoblast (arrow) showing 'halo' artefact. Giemsa.

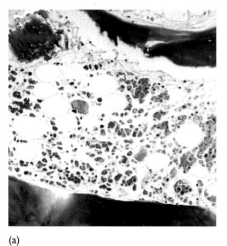

(a)

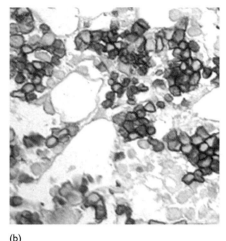

(b)

Fig 2.18 Neonatal marrow showing erythroid colonies which should not be confused with metastatic disease. (a) Giemsa. (b) Immunostaining for red cell glycophorin. APAAP.

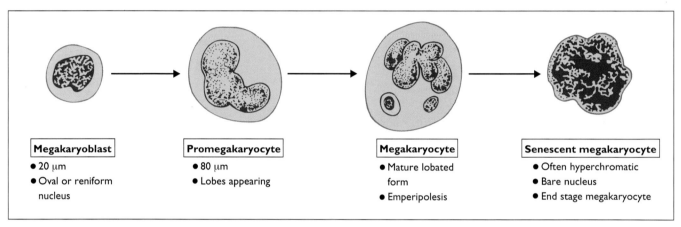

Megakaryoblast
- 20 μm
- Oval or reniform nucleus

Promegakaryocyte
- 80 μm
- Lobes appearing

Megakaryocyte
- Mature lobated form
- Emperipolesis

Senescent megakaryocyte
- Often hyperchromatic
- Bare nucleus
- End stage megakaryocyte

Fig 2.19 Schematic illustration of megakaryocytic differentiation.

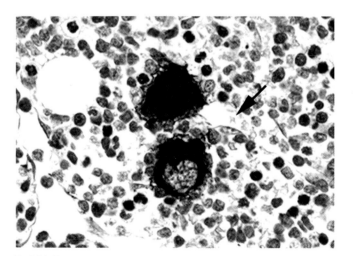

Fig 2.20 Two megakaryocytes immunostained for CD61 lying in close proximity to a venous sinusoid (arrow). APAAP.

Table 2.2 Causes of erythroid hyperplasia.

Peripheral red cell loss or destruction
    e.g. haemorrhage
    e.g. haemolytic anaemia
Ineffective erythropoiesis
    e.g. red cell membrane defects
    e.g. abnormal haemoglobin
    e.g. nutritional deficiency
Administration of erythropoietin

Table 2.3 Megakaryocyte morphology in haematological conditions.

Condition	Megakaryocyte morphology
Reactive	Emperipolesis
Idiopathic thrombocytopaenic purpura	Increased numbers of small immature megakaryocytes
Myelodysplastic syndrome	Increased numbers of small (micro) megakaryocytes, diffusely arranged
Chronic myeloid leukaemia	Increased numbers of small (micro) megakaryocytes, diffuse, small clusters
Essential thrombocythaemia	Increased numbers of giant megakaryocytes, often in clusters
Polycythaemia rubra vera	Increased numbers of pleomorphic megakaryocytes, all sizes, clustered
Primary myelofibrosis	Increased numbers of pleomorphic megakaryocytes, all sizes, clustered

Table 2.4 A comparison of the features which may help discriminate between benign lymphoid aggregates in bone marrow and neoplastic involvement.

Benign	Neoplastic
Rounded aggregates	May be irregular
Well circumscribed regular small lymphocytes	Cellular atypia may be present
Elderly population	Wide age range
< 3 mm in diameter	May be > 3 mm diameter
Never paratrabecular	May be paratrabecular
Germinal centres (5% of cases)	No germinal centres
May contain plasma cells and eosinophils	Usually just lymphoid cells
Polyclonal light chain expression	Monoclonal light chain pattern
1–3 aggregates per trephine	> 3 aggregates per trephine

Table 2.5 Causes of a reactive plasmacytosis.

HIV
Hepatitis
Systemic lupus erythematosis
Rheumatoid arthritis
Iron and folate deficiency
Alcohol abuse
Hodgkin's disease

Table 2.6 A comparison of the histological features of reactive plasmacytosis and multiple myeloma.

Reactive plasmacytosis	Multiple myeloma
Majority are mature plasma cells	Variation in size and differentiation, intermediate forms common
Nucleoli uncommon	Nucleoli often present
No clusters	Clusters common
Single layer around capillaries	Several cells deep around capillaries

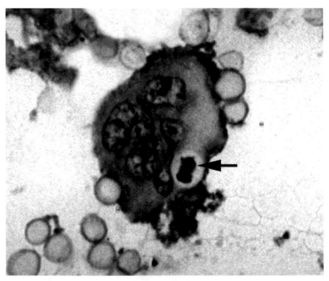

Fig 2.21 Megakaryocyte showing emperipolesis. A neutrophil (arrow) is present within the megakaryocyte. Giemsa.

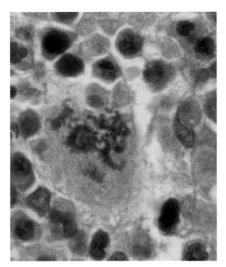

Fig 2.22 Megakaryocyte showing mitosis. H&E.

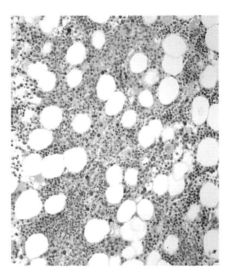

Fig 2.23 Distribution of B cells (immuno-staining for CD79a) in normal marrow. Immunoperoxidase.

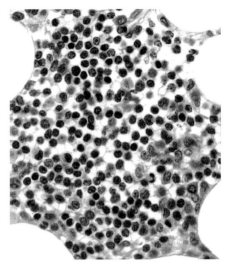

Fig 2.24 Reactive lymphoid nodule in normal marrow. H&E.

It should be remembered that in a histological section one is seeing only a small part of a megakaryocyte and in order to obtain a reliable impression of megakaryocyte morphology many megakaryocytes should be examined. Emperipolesis (the safe passage of intact cells through the cytoplasm of another cell) is occasionally seen to occur in megakaryocytes. Although its significance is not known it is seen more frequently in reactive conditions and appears to be a non-specific feature (Fig. 2.21). Occasionally, megakaryocytes may be seen in mitosis (Fig. 2.22).

The term, 'pleomorphism', is used to describe megakaryocytes in a number of diseases, particularly the myeloproliferative disorders. Since normal megakaryocytes exhibit polyploidy there is an inevitable degree of nuclear pleomorphism in these cells. None the less, for diagnostic purposes, some megakaryocytes can be described as pleomorphic, in a pathological sense, when variations in cell size, shape, nuclear morphology and topographical distribution exceed that seen in a normal marrow. Table 2.3 gives a summary of these changes.

Other cells

A number of other cell types, which are not directly related to the haematopoietic tissues, can be identified on tissue sections. These include lymphocytes, plasma cells, mast cells and macrophages.

LYMPHOCYTES

Normal adult marrow contains an inconspicuous population of both B and T lymphocytes throughout the marrow (Fig. 2.23). They may occur as small aggregates (Fig. 2.24). These lymphoid aggregates increase in number with age, being frequently seen in the elderly population. If there are more than three lymphoid aggregates per trephine, it does suggest a neoplastic rather than a reactive process. Distinguishing between benign lymphoid aggregates and those which are neoplastic can be difficult and their significance remains unresolved (Table 2.4).[2-4]

Demonstration of monoclonality using light chain immuno-staining may be possible in a number of cases, although this does not mean that the patient will subsequently develop the clinical features of a lymphoma. This may be partly because many of these patients are elderly and will die of unrelated conditions.

In neonates the normal marrow contains a much increased number of lymphocytes, which may account for up to 50% of the marrow's cellularity.

PLASMA CELLS

These are easily identified in normal adult marrow and form about 2% of the cell population in the marrow. They may occur singly, in small groups (2–3 cells) or more commonly in association with capillaries where they form a single layer around the vessel (Fig. 2.6). Immature and binucleate forms are uncommon. Plasma cells with intracytoplasmic accumulations of immunoglobulin, i.e. Russell bodies, may be found in both reactive and malignant plasma cells.

It is difficult, using morphological criteria alone, to differentiate between a highly reactive plasmacytosis (Table 2.5) and a well-differentiated myeloma, since both conditions may display large numbers of plasma cells (Table 2.6).

Assessment of light chain expression is easily performed in wax-embedded specimens and is a valuable means of differentiating between these two conditions since myeloma will display light chain restriction.

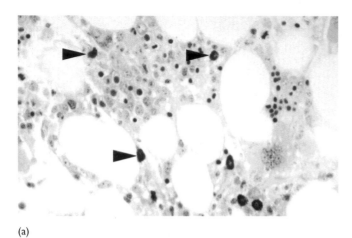

(a)

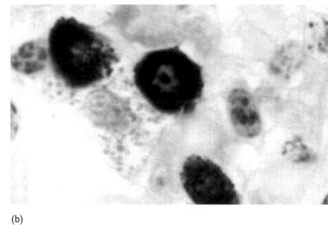

(b)

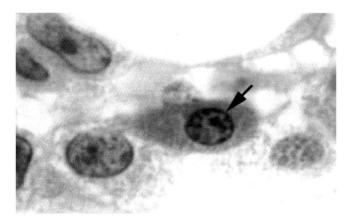

(c)

Fig 2.25. (a) A low power view of normal marrow showing scattered mast cells (arrowheads). (b) and (c) High power views showing (b) how Giemsa staining highlights mast cells which are often difficult to identify on (c) H&E (arrow).

Table 2.7 Causes of mast cell hyperplasia.

Lymphoproliferative disease, particularly Waldenström's macroglobulinaemia
Alcohol excess
Radiation

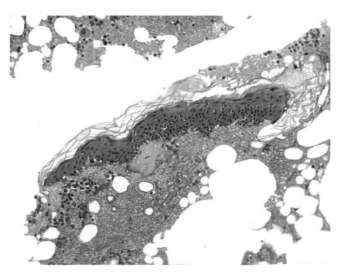

Fig 2.26 Fragment of epidermis introduced into the marrow during the biopsy procedures.

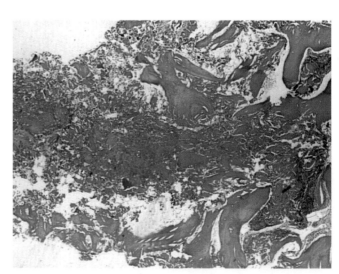

Fig 2.27 Bone dust filling the marrow cavity is an artefact of trephining. H&E.

Human immunodeficiency virus (HIV) infection

Chapter 3

Introduction

HIV infection may result in many changes to the bone marrow. These include reactive processes, secondary infections and the development of malignancies. They are a consequence of the virus's ability to impair the body's immune system. Some of the changes may be seen at a relatively early stage of HIV infection, before the onset of full-blown AIDS (Acquired Immune Deficiency Syndrome).

Clinical features

Within developed countries AIDS is predominantly associated with homosexuals and intravenous drug abusers and does not appear to have spread significantly into the heterosexual population as is the case in the Third World countries.

Consequently most patients in this country (UK) with HIV-related disease are young or middle-aged and male. They may present with a wide variety of complaints, the most common of which include weight loss, lymphadenopathy, diarrhoea, oral thrush, cough, skin problems and general weakness. Aspiration of the marrow can be difficult.

Histopathology of the bone marrow

Bone marrow changes are common in HIV-related disease. The cellularity is usually increased (Fig. 3.1) although approximately 20% of cases are hypocellular (Fig. 3.2).

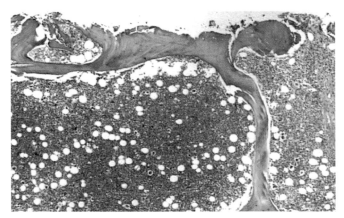

Fig 3.1 Typical hypercellular marrow seen in uncomplicated HIV infection. H&E.

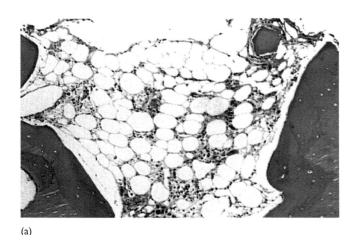

(a)

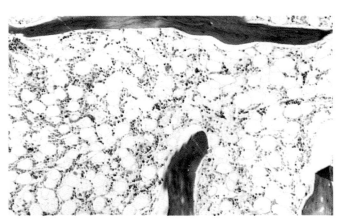

(b)

Fig 3.2 Examples of hypocellularity seen in HIV infection. (a) H&E. (b) Giemsa.

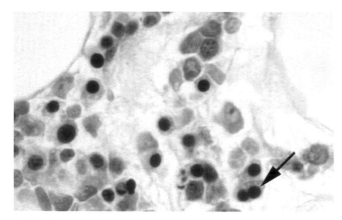

Fig 3.3 Dyserythropoiesis in HIV infection. Binucleate normoblast (arrow). Giemsa.

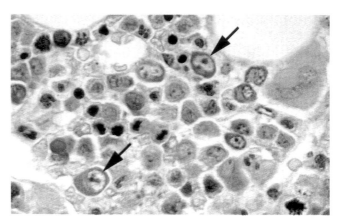

Fig 3.4 Megaloblastic precursors (arrows) in HIV infection. Giemsa.

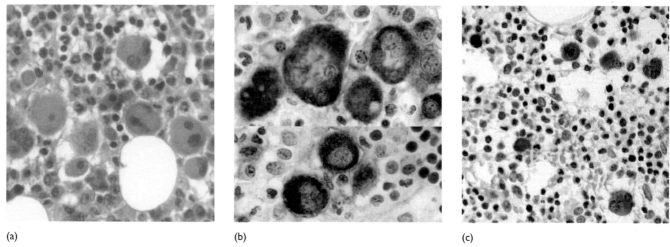

(a)

(b)

(c)

Fig 3.5 Micromegakaryocytes in HIV infection. (a) Giemsa. (b) CD31. (c) CD61.

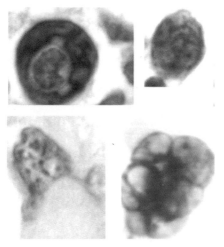

Fig 3.6 Naked megakaryocyte nuclei. Giemsa.

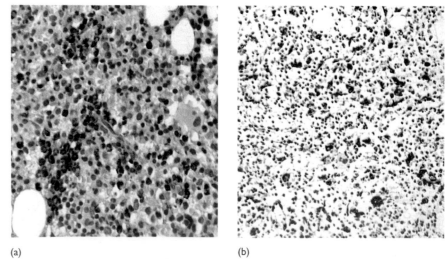

(a)

(b)

Fig 3.7 Increased numbers of plasma cells. (a) Antibody VS38 and macrophages. (b) Antibody against CD68 in HIV-infected marrow.

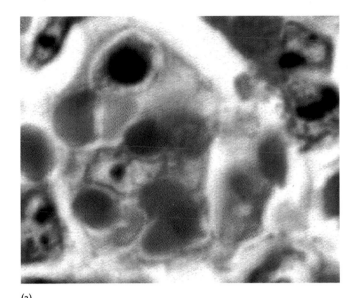

(a)

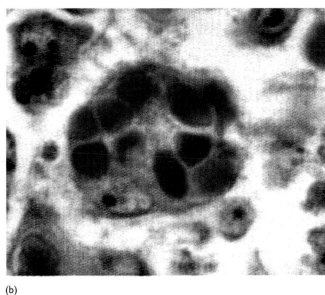

(b)

Fig 3.8 Macrophages demonstrating erythrophagocytosis. Giemsa.

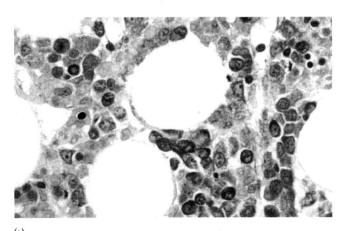

(a)

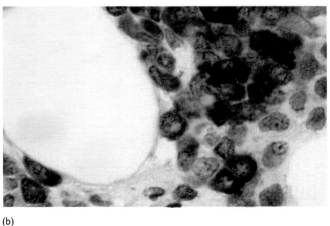

(b)

Fig 3.9 Increased numbers of plasma cells. (a) Giemsa. (b) Antibody VS38.

Reactive features

Up to three-quarters of HIV-infected marrow show dyshaematopoiesis with myelodysplastic-like features affecting all three cell lines. Members of the granulocyte series may show nuclear abnormalities and decreased granularity. Eosinophilia is common (seen in 15% of cases). The erythroid series may show abnormalities of normoblast nuclei, especially binucleate forms and irregular nuclear outlines (Fig. 3.3) and occasionally megaloblastoid change is seen (Fig. 3.4).

The latter feature is said to be more common in patients taking Zidovudine (AZT) where increased numbers of proerythroblasts with megaloblastic features are present. The megakaryocyte series shows increased numbers of micromegakaryocytes and mono-nuclear forms (Fig. 3.5).

Naked megakaryocyte nuclei are also seen and probably represent platelet-depleted (i.e. end stage) megakaryocytes (Fig. 3.6). In addition to abnormalities involving haematopoietic tissue, considerable alterations to the stromal environment may also occur. Contributing to the hypercellularity of HIV-infected marrows are increased numbers of plasma cells, lymphocytes and macrophages (Fig. 3.7). Some of the latter may display erythrophagocytosis (Fig. 3.8).

The plasmacytosis can be particularly striking (Fig. 3.9) and easily mistaken for multiple myeloma. However, the plasma cells are polyclonal in nature, as demonstrated by light chain immunostaining. Aggregates of lymphocytes are not infrequent. Focal lesions consisting of loose, ill-defined aggregates of lymphoid cells, histiocytes and associated vascular proliferation may be seen and are

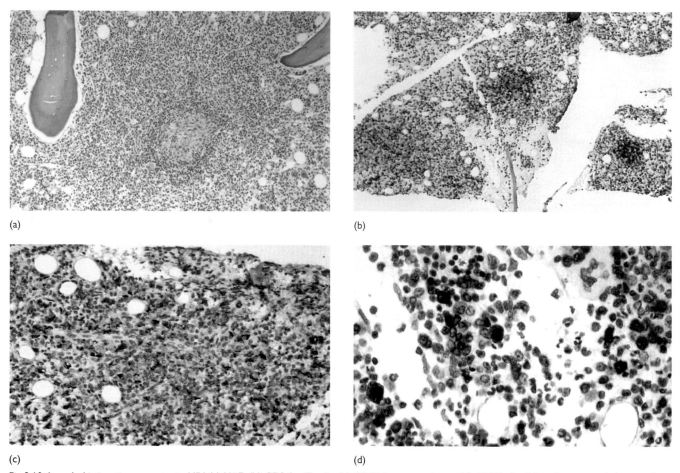

(a)

(b)

(c)

(d)

Fig 3.10 Lymphohistiocytic aggregates in HIV. (a) H&E. (b) CD3 for T cells. (c) CD68 for macrophages. (d) CD79a for B lymphocytes and plasma cells.

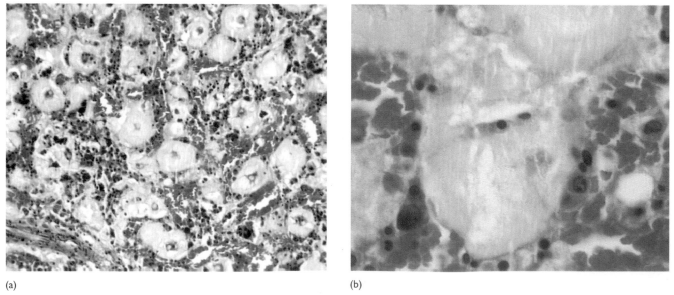

(a)

(b)

Fig 3.11 Serous atrophy in HIV. (a) Low power. (b) High power. Both H&E.

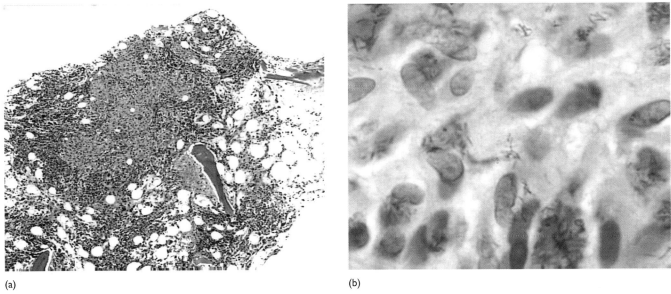

(a)

(b)

Fig 3.12 Granuloma in TB infected HIV marrow. (a) H&E. (b) ZN for tubercle bacilli.

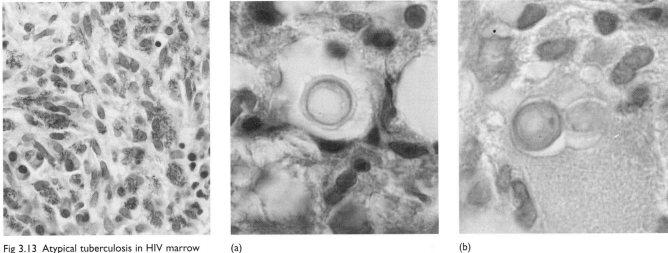

Fig 3.13 Atypical tuberculosis in HIV marrow not associated with granulomata. ZN stain.

(a)

(b)

Fig 3.14 HIV-associated cryptococcal infection. (a) H&E. (b) Mucicarmine.

known as lymphohistiocytic aggregates resembling those lesions seen in angioimmunoblastic lymphoadenopathy (AILD) (Fig. 3.10). Conventional granulomas may be found in the absence of any obvious aetiology.

Serous atrophy (gelatinous transformation) is frequently seen and when extensive the appearance is striking (Fig. 3.11). It is usually associated with more severe HIV-related disease which has involved rapid weight loss.

Secondary infections

These are common and patients often have multiple infections. The most commonly encountered are those involving acid-fast bacilli, usually tubercle bacillus (TB) or *Mycobacterium avium intracellulare* complex (MAIC). Granulomas are usually present in marrows infected by these organisms, although this is not always the case (Fig. 3.12). It is prudent to stain all known HIV marrow biopsies (and indeed all types of tissue biopsies from HIV-infected patients) with a ZN stain, whether granulomas are present or not. The number of bacilli seen may vary considerably although large numbers are often present (Fig. 3.13).

The fungi *Cryptococcus* (Fig. 3.14) and *Histoplasma* (Fig. 3.15) and the protozoan Leishmania (Fig. 3.16) are usually found in reactive macrophages often associated with granuloma formation (Fig. 3.17). CMV infection may be detected by characteristic nuclear

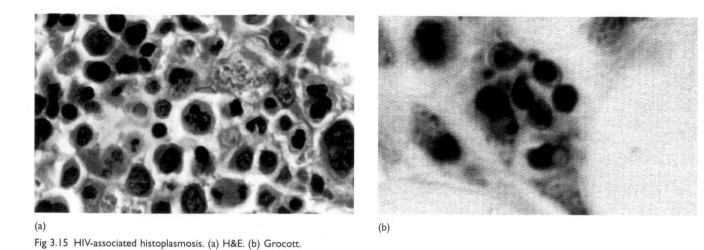

(a)

(b)

Fig 3.15 HIV-associated histoplasmosis. (a) H&E. (b) Grocott.

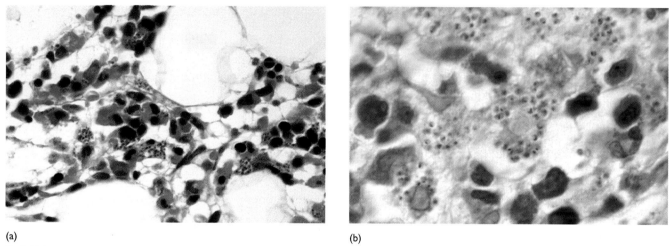

(a)

(b)

Fig 3.16 *Leishmania donovani* bodies in macrophage cytoplasm. (a) H&E. (b) Giemsa.

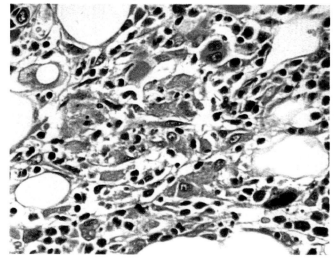

Fig 3.17 Histoplasmosis associated with granuloma formation. H&E.

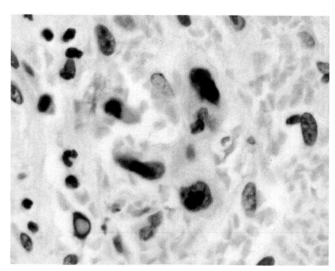

Fig 3.18 CMV infection. Immunoperoxidase.

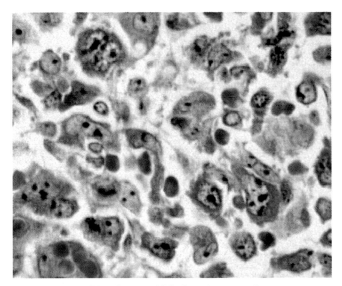

Fig 3.19 Large cell lymphoma in HIV-infected marrow. Giemsa.

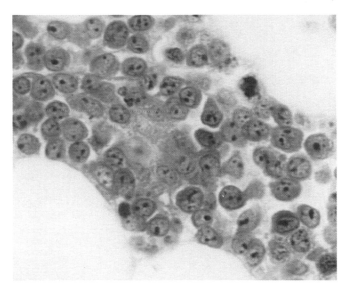

Fig 3.20 (a)

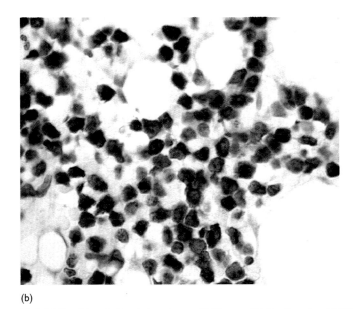

(b)

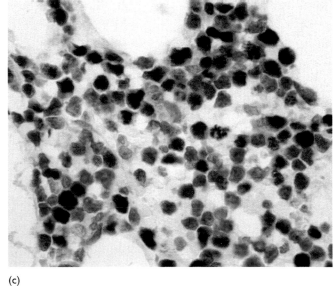

(c)

Fig 3.20 B cell lymphoblastic lymphoma. (a) Giemsa. (b) B cell marker CD79a with high proliferation index. (c) Immunoperoxidase for proliferation associated marker JC1.

inclusions, particularly within endothelial cells (Fig. 3.18). *Pneumocystis carinii* infection need not necessarily remain within the lungs and can become systemic, occasionally involving the bone marrow.[1]

Malignancies

Patients with HIV infection have an increased risk of developing a non-Hodgkin's lymphoma. These are high-grade malignancies and often involve the marrow. They are usually of a B cell immunophenotype and have a large cell (centroblastic or immunoblastic) (Fig. 3.19) or lymphoblastic morphology (Fig. 3.20).

Hodgkin's disease also appears to be increased in HIV-infected individuals (Fig. 3.21) and may have a more aggressive course than the conventional type.

Kaposi's sarcoma can involve most organs including, rarely, the bone marrow (Table 3.1).

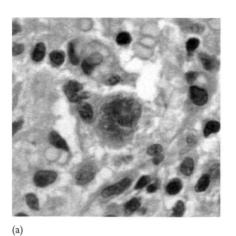

(a)

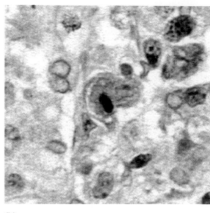

(b)

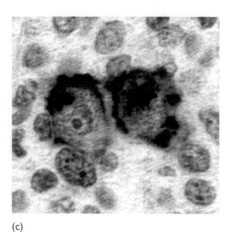

(c)

Fig 3.21 Hodgkin's disease in HIV-infected marrow. (a) H&E. (b) Giemsa. (c) CD30 immunostain.

Myelodysplastic-like features	Stromal features
Seen in 75%	Increased plasma cells and macrophages
All three cell lines affected	Macrophages showing erythrophagocytosis
15% have eosinophilia	Serous atrophy
Megaloblastoid features	Lymphocytosis
Nuclear abnormalities in normoblasts	Lymphohistiocytic aggregates (AILD-like lesions)
Nuclear abnormalities and decreased granularity in myeloid series	Vascular proliferation
Micromegakaryocytes	
Mononuclear megakaryocytes	
Naked megakaryocyte nuclei	
Infections	**Malignancies**
Leishmaniasis	Kaposi's sarcoma
Pneumocystis carinii	Non-Hodgkin's lymphoma
Cryptococcus neoformans	Hodgkin's disease
Histoplasma capsulatum	
Mycobacterium avium intracellulare	
CMV	
TB	

Table 3.1 Summary of features seen in HIV-positive bone marrow biopsies.

Diagnostic problems

1 Misdiagnosis as MDS is unlikely since there are usually other features to suggest HIV infection. In addition, the clinical features including the patient's age would be unusual for a diagnosis of MDS.
2 A striking plasmacytosis may provide confusion with multiple myeloma. Immunohistochemistry will resolve this by demonstrating that the plasma cell population is polyclonal.
3 Megaloblastoid change seen in members of the erythroid series should not be misdiagnosed as leukaemia or megaloblastic anaemia, since the change is accompanied by other features of HIV infection.
4 Distinction between secondary infection by TB and by MAIC may be possible since MAIC tends to be PAS positive in addition to being ZN positive.

Summary of key points
- Perform a ZN stain on all known HIV-infected marrow biopsies.
- HIV infection may cause a number of histological changes, none of which are specific.
- Consider HIV infection in any marrow which shows ill-defined abnormalities which are not diagnostic of other conditions.

Reference

1 Telsak EE, Cote RJ, Gold JMW, Campbell SW, Armstrong D. Extrapulmonary *Pneumocystis carinii* infections. *Rev Infect Dis* 1990; **12**: 380–386.

Anaemias and aplasias

Chapter 4

ANAEMIAS

Introduction

The majority of anaemias are diagnosed and treated by a wide range of clinicians with only the more severe or complicated needing specialist haematological attention. Even then only a minority of these cases come to trephine biopsy. This reduces the pathologist's experience in these areas which can lead to a misdiagnosis. This can be overcome to some extent by persuading the haematologist to submit the particles remaining after bone marrow aspiration for histopathology, even if no trephine is taken.

The evaluation of marrow iron stores is an important consideration in the diagnosis of many anaemias. This can be assessed on lightly decalcified sections processed promptly to paraffin and well stained by Giemsa, though one should be aware that some iron loss may occur during decalcification.

Iron deficiency anaemia

Haematologists rarely examine the bone marrow in iron deficiency so that when trephines are taken they are often complicated by other clinical conditions. In uncomplicated iron deficiency anaemia the marrow is usually slightly hypercellular due to increased erythropoiesis. Iron stores are reduced or absent (Fig. 4.1).

Anaemia of chronic disease

Again trephines are not a first line of investigation in the anaemias of chronic infections, inflammatory diseases or malignancy. The cellularity is normal or slightly reduced with iron detectable in macrophages (though many of these patients will have had blood transfusions) (Fig. 4.2).

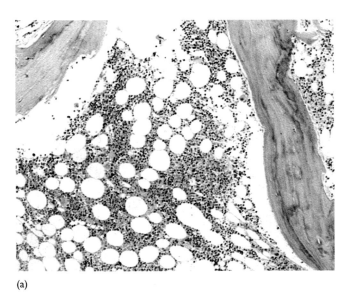

(a)

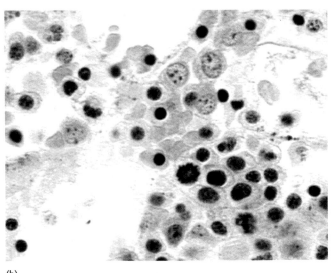

(b)

Fig 4.1 Iron deficiency anaemia. (a) Hypercellular marrow showing (b) increased erythropoiesis. Giemsa.

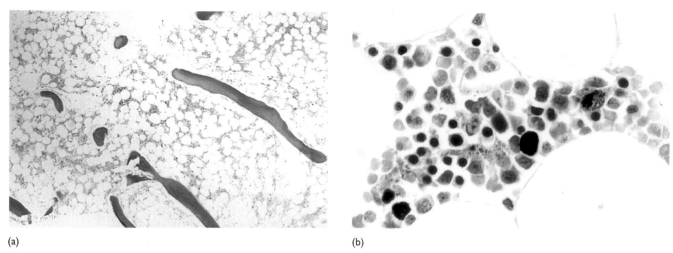

(a)

(b)

Fig 4.2 Anaemia of chronic disease. (a) Normal cellularity for age. (b) Iron in macrophages (green). Giemsa.

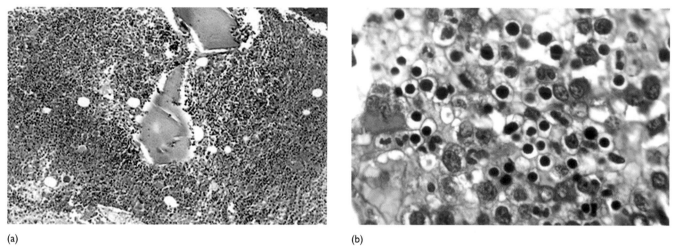

(a)

(b)

Fig 4.3 Autoimmune haemolytic anaemia. (a) Hypercellular marrow. (b) Erythroid hyperplasia. Giemsa.

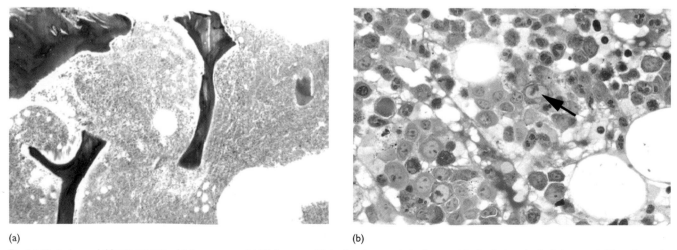

(a)

(b)

Fig 4.4 Typical megaloblastic anaemia. (a) Low power. (b) High power. Note the characteristic elongated 'coin slot' nucleoli of the megaloblasts (arrow) and metamyelocytes (arrowhead). Giemsa.

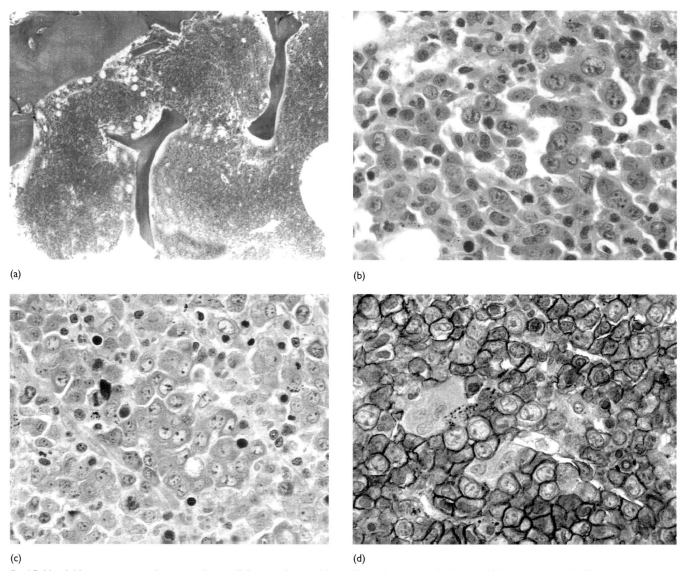

(a)

(b)

(c)

(d)

Fig 4.5 Megaloblastic anaemia with extreme hypercellularity with many blast cells simulating acute leukaemia. (a) Low power. H&E. (b) High power. H&E. (c) High power. Giemsa. (d) Immunostain for red cell glycophorin. Peroxidase.

Haemolytic anaemia

A trephine is usually taken to exclude an underlying malignancy such as CLL. Uncomplicated haemolytic marrows are hypercellular with marked erythroid hyperplasia but little else of note (Fig. 4.3).

Megaloblastic anaemia

The marrow is usually hypercellular with loss of fat cells including the first fat space around the bone. The marrow is dominated by erythroid hyperplasia with significant left shifting including the characteristic megaloblastic erythroid precursors. This and the cellular-

ity may be so marked that it could be misdiagnosed as a malignancy such as leukaemia, lymphoma or even carcinoma. This is easier to do on an H&E since the deep blue cytoplasm of a good Giemsa often gives the game away. The other cell lines also demonstrate changes, most notably giant metamyelocytes in the granulocyte series. Megakaryocytes are smaller, slightly increased in numbers and may have hyperlobated nuclei. These changes are typically caused by B12 or folate deficiency, although a number of drugs affecting DNA synthesis have also been implicated (Figs 4.4 and 4.5).

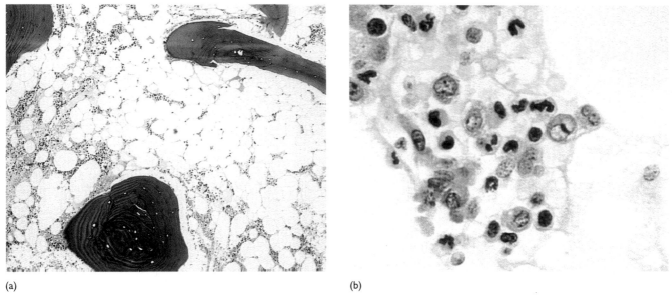

(a)   (b)

Fig 4.6 Drug-induced macrocytosis. (a) Low power. (b) High power. Giemsa.

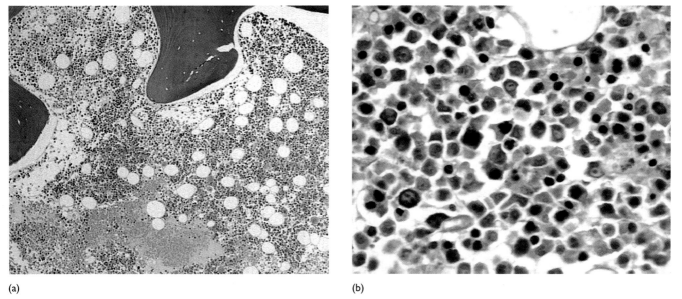

(a)   (b)

Fig 4.7 Congenital dyserythropoietic anaemia in a child's marrow. (a) Low power. (b) High power showing disrupted erythroid colonies with marked pleomorphic features in all cell types. Giemsa.

Table 4.1 Drugs which may cause aplasia.

Type of drug	Example
Antibiotic	Chloramphenicol
Anti-inflammatory	Phenylbutazone
Anti-epileptics	Phenytoin
Anti-malarials	Mepacrine
Anti-diabetic	Chlorpropamide

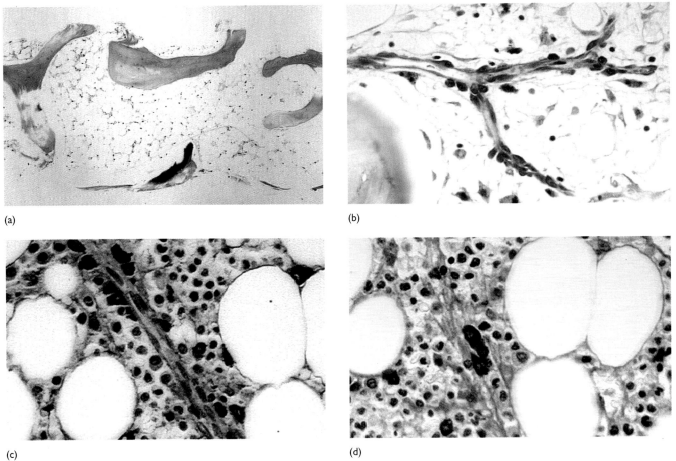

(a)

(b)

(c)

(d)

Fig 4.8 Aplastic anaemia. (a) Low power. Giemsa. (b) Vessel surrounded by reactive plasma cells showing polyclonal light chain production. (c) Kappa immunostain. (d) Lambda immunostain.

Other macrocytic anaemias with many causes including drugs and alcohol can give rise to megaloblastic changes. The cellularity is usually normal or low without the dramatic picture of true megaloblastic anaemia (Fig. 4.6).

Congenital dyserythropoietic anaemias

These are very rare inherited conditions which usually do not include a biopsy in their evaluation. The trephine is hypercellular, often with marked dyserythropoiesis and should always be considered in the differential diagnosis of dyserythropoiesis in children (Fig. 4.7).

APLASIAS

It is not easy to find a good definition for bone marrow aplasia. Possibly the best approach is to consider it a clinicopathological correlation of profound cellular hypoplasia combined with pancytopaenia. Fibrosis and malignant infiltration are usually excluded as causes.

Aplastic anaemia will result from chemotherapy or wide field radiotherapy; the effect is dose related and inevitable. Many drugs can give rise to aplasia (Table 4.1) as will a variety of viral infections, especially hepatitis B. In a proportion of cases no obvious cause (often referred to as idiopathic cases) can be identified. Many of these are suspected to be hypocellular myelodysplastic syndromes and indeed there is evidence that something like 10% of long-term survivors of aplastic anaemia will go on to develop AML.[1]

Aplastic anaemias

The trephine features are similar regardless of the cause. The marrow is profoundly hypocellular though often focal areas of slightly increased cellularity may be seen. Inspection of these areas is often disappointing as they largely consist of inflammatory and stromal cells (Fig. 4.8).

It is of course important to exclude hypocellular MDS/AML by ensuring that clusters of blast cells are not overlooked. With recovery which may require steroid or growth factor treatment in

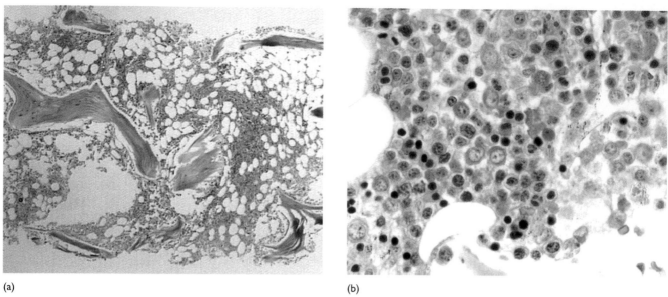

(a)

(b)

Fig 4.9 (a) Marrow appearances one year after successful treatment for typical aplastic anaemia. (b) High power view shows dysplastic changes (reduced granulocyte differentiation, dyserythropoiesis) which should not be interpreted as preleukaemic. Giemsa.

idiosyncratic cases there is frequently a period when the marrow appears profoundly dysplastic. One should be careful not to over-interpret this since given time the marrow will revert to a healthy state, especially in the post-chemotherapy, viral- or drug-induced cases (Fig. 4.9).

Reference

1 Gordon-Smith EC, Weatherall DJ, Ledingham JGG, Warrell DA (eds). Aplastic anaemia and other causes of bone marrow failure. *Oxford Textbook of Medicine* 3rd edition. Oxford University Press. Oxford, 1996.

The myelodysplastic syndromes Chapter 5

Introduction

A preleukaemic state has been recognized for some time although different nomenclatures, e.g. 'smouldering leukaemia', 'preleukaemic syndrome' and 'dysmyelopoietic syndrome', have given rise to some confusion. This situation has, to some extent, been clarified by the French–American–British (FAB) co-operative group who in 1982 proposed the term 'myelodysplasia' and defined five subtypes.[1]

These are:

1 refractory anaemia (RA);
2 refractory anaemia with ringed sideroblasts (RARS);
3 refractory anaemia with excess of blasts (RAEB);
4 chronic myelomonocytic leukaemia (CMML);
5 refractory anaemia with excess of blasts in transformation (RAEBt).

Although myelodysplasia is commonly thought of as preleukaemic it should not be forgotten that most leukaemias, particularly in children and young adults, develop de novo.

It should be emphasized that the FAB classification was designed to be used by haematologists not histopathologists and is not directly applicable to tissue sections where certain features are not apparent. For example, it is rarely possible to identify ringed sideroblasts in histological sections of trephine biopsies.*

The inclusion of CMML as part of MDS is not universally accepted. Some authorities argue that it should be considered as an established leukaemia and be placed with the myeloproliferative disorders.[2,3]

Trephine biopsy plays an important part in the diagnosis of MDS and in monitoring its evolution, particularly when a dry tap is obtained (partly because the marrow is hypercellular and partly because of an increase in reticulin fibres). In addition, the histology provides information not available from a smear preparation, such as topographical abnormalities and changes to the marrow stroma.

---

* These are erythroblasts with a ring of mitochondrial-associated free iron distributed around the nucleus and are probably related to the abnormal erythropoiesis seen in MDS.

Myelodysplasia (MDS)
Clinical features

The typical picture is of an elderly patient (median 65 years) complaining of bleeding, recurrent infections or tiredness. They have an anaemia which is unresponsive to iron supplements. Hepato-splenomegaly and lymphadenopathy are not typical. The clinical course is variable; some patients progress to AML whilst others require little in the way of treatment. The majority of patients die from haemorrhage or sepsis.

The average survival for each group in the FAB classification is:

RA	60 months
RARS	30 months
CMML	15 months
RAEB & RAEBt	10 months

Histopathology of the bone marrow

The appearances of MDS in tissue sections of the marrow consist mainly of loss of cellular differentiation and disruption of normal architecture. These changes can be considered analogous to those seen in premalignant conditions affecting other organs, e.g. cervical intraepithelial neoplasia, adenomatous polyps of the bowel and actinic keratoses. MDS is a stem cell disorder so that abnormalities may be apparent in any of the three blood-forming cell lines. It is a common misconception that marked abnormalities must be detected in each cell line in order to diagnose MDS on trephine sections. In fact the identifiable abnormalities may be restricted to only one series, e.g. the erythroid in sideroblastic anaemia.

CELLULARITY

The marrow is hypercellular in the majority of cases (80%). In the remainder the marrow is normocellular or even hypocellular.

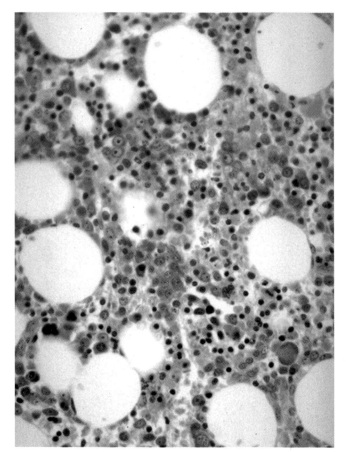

Fig 5.1 Typical jumbled appearance of cell types in myelodysplasia. Giemsa.

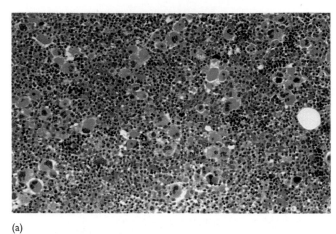

(a)

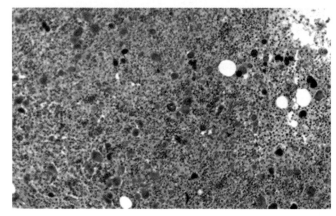

(b)

Fig 5.2 Increased numbers of megakaryocytes in MDS. (a) Seen by H&E. (b) Highlighted by immunostaining for CD61.

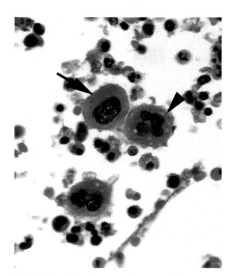

Fig 5.3 Typical micromegakaryocyte (arrow-head) next to a monolobated form (arrow) in MDS. H&E.

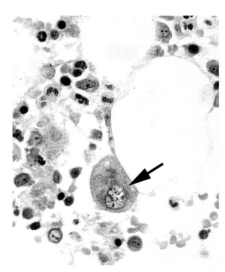

Fig 5.4 Monolobated megakaryocyte (arrow) in MDS. Giemsa.

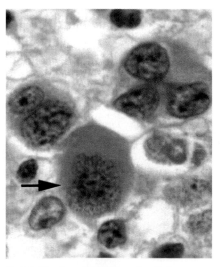

Fig 5.5 Megakaryoblast (arrow) with 2 micromegakaryocytes. H&E.

ABNORMALITIES OF MARROW ARCHITECTURE

The most striking feature seen at low power is the disruption of the normal cellular distribution. The appearance is of all cell lines randomly mixed together. The marrow stroma is also altered. Oedema, extravasation of red blood cells, sinus ectasia, increased reticulin formation, haemosiderin-laden macrophages, plasmacytosis and lymphoid aggregate formation all add to the anarchic appearance of MDS (Fig. 5.1). To appreciate these changes it is essential to have a knowledge of normal marrow histology.

DYSMEGAKARYOPOIESIS

The number of megakaryocytes is increased, which is best demonstrated immunohistochemically (Fig. 5.2). Their distribution is abnormal, with many having a paratrabecular location. A number of abnormalities in size, shape and nuclear lobe configuration may be present.

1 *Micromegakaryocytes.* These are normal in appearance except that the diameter of the cell is much reduced (Fig. 5.3).

2 *Monolobated megakaryocytes* (Fig. 5.4). These are not to be confused with megakaryoblasts which are normal precursors seen in a number of reactive conditions. Monolobated megakaryocytes are larger (>30 μm) than megakaryoblasts, have more cytoplasm (similar in amount to mature megakaryocytes) and a single lobed nucleus without nucleoli. They are reported to be in increased numbers (>50%) in cases of MDS showing a deletion of all or part of chromosome 5q (the so called 5q minus syndrome[4]). This is of clinical relevance because patients with the 5q- syndrome have a lower incidence of leukaemic transformation.

3 *Megakaryoblasts* (Fig. 5.5). These are increased in number and may be dysplastic. They are small, have a high nuclear/cytoplasmic ratio and the nuclei are hypolobated and may have nucleoli.

4 *Topographical abnormalities.* The main abnormalities are their paratrabecular distribution and clustering of two or more megakaryocytes with direct cellular contact ('kissing').

DYSERYTHROPOIESIS

This is characterized by enlarged irregular erythroid colonies containing increased numbers of immature cells. These colonies lack the symmetry and central localization seen in normal marrows. These features may be highlighted by immunocytochemical staining for red cell antigens (Fig. 5.6). Frequently the immature precursors are clustered together and are separated from the more differentiated erythroid cells by other marrow elements. Cytological abnormalities include binucleate or irregularly shaped normoblasts and megaloblastic precursors (Fig. 5.7).

DYSGRANULOPOIESIS

A reduction in granulocytic maturation is usually evident though other abnormalities are less impressive than in the other cell series.

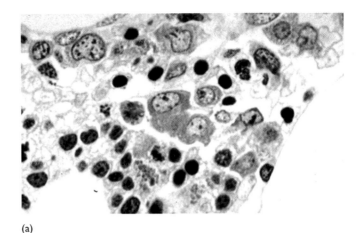

(a)

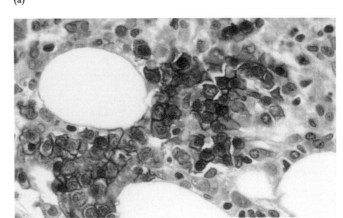

(b)

Fig 5.6 Enlarged irregular erythroid colony in MDS highlighted by immunostaining for glycophorin C. (a) Giemsa. (b) Immunoperoxidase.

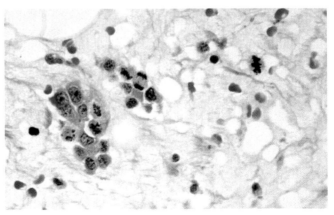

Fig 5.7 Clusters of immature erythroid precursors in MDS. Giemsa.

Reduced cytoplasmic granulation and abnormalities of nuclear lobation are best appreciated in smear preparations.

Abnormally located immature precursors (ALIP)

ALIPs are generally believed to represent primitive myeloid (i.e. granulocytic) precursors (Fig. 5.8). They are abnormal because of their location in the middle of the marrow and also because they occur in groups. They were reported to indicate a poorer prognosis because of a higher association with leukaemic transformation.

This is a controversial area with strong advocates[5,6] and sceptics.[7–9] Part of the difficulty in resolving this dilemma lies in the subjective criteria for the recognition of ALIPs. Consequently there is no current consensus on their value in diagnosis.

Histological correlation with the FAB classification

There is only a limited correlation between the histological findings in MDS and the separate categories recognized by the FAB classification. In general, a low blast cell count correlates with RA and RARS whereas with an increase in the number of blast cells the syndrome is more likely to be RAEB or RAEBt. Immunohistochemistry, using QBEND10 (CD34) to highlight blast cells, may be of use in identifying cases of RAEB and RAEBt.[10]

Chronic myelomonocytic leukaemia (CMML)
Clinical features

Clinical features include anaemia, hepatosplenomegaly and, occasionally, skin infiltrates. The clinical course is usually protracted although transformation to an acute leukaemia may occur.

Diagnosis

The diagnosis is usually made on the marrow aspirate and peripheral blood examination. The peripheral blood monocyte count is > 1x10⁹/l (of which < 5% are blasts). The marrow is hypercellular with < 20% blasts.

Histopathology of the bone marrow

The appearances seen in most trephines are those of a myeloproliferative disorder and changes indicative of myelodysplasia are usually absent. The cytological appearances are characteristically those of a leukaemic infiltration of the marrow by cells showing a variable differentiation between granulocytes and monocytes (the so-called myelomonocyte) (Fig 5.9). Immunocytochemical demonstration of myeloid and monocytic antigens may be helpful in confirming the diagnosis.

Diagnostic problems
Differential diagnosis

Other diseases can produce a myelodysplastic-like picture in the marrow. Hairy cell leukaemia and HIV infection are two of the commonest examples which have been considered in other chapters.

Distinction between MDS, acute leukaemia and aplastic anaemia in marrows which are hypocellular is difficult. Another diagnostic problem is the separation of RAEBt and CML in accelerated phase.

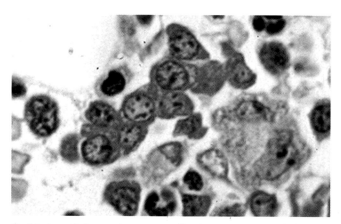

Fig 5.8 A small cluster of precursor cells of uncertain origin which the authors believe represent ALIPs. Giemsa.

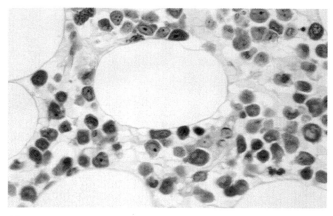

(a)

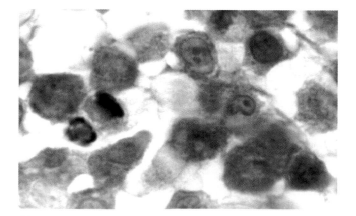

(b)

Fig 5.9 In CMML the marrow is hypercellular and is characterized by an increased number of myelocytes with a lack of more mature granulocytes (a & b). Giemsa.

Areas such as these can rarely be resolved by histology alone and emphasize the need for close clinical correlations.

Secondary MDS

MDS may follow the use of chemotherapy or radiotherapy, for example in the treatment of Hodgkin's disease or myeloma. Secondary MDS, like primary MDS, may progress to AML. The marrow is often hypocellular and dyserythropoiesis is a prominent feature.

Overlap between myelodysplasia and myeloproliferation

In a minority of cases it may not be possible on histological criteria alone to make a definite diagnosis of myelodysplasia or myeloproliferation. This reflects the fact that there are no absolute histological features pathognomonic for either condition. Clinical details and cytogenetic studies will only resolve some of these cases. This has led to a view that myelodysplasia and myeloproliferation are a spectrum of myeloid neoplasia rather than separate entities.

References

1 Bennett JM, Catovsky D, Daniel MT, Flandrin G, Galton DAG, Gralnick HR, Sultan C. The French–American–British (FAB) co-operation group. Proposals for the classification of myelodysplastic syndromes. *Br J Haematol* 1982; **51**: 189–199.

2 Frisch B and Bartl R. Bone marrow histology in myelodysplastic syndromes. *Scand J Haematol* 1986; **Suppl 45**: 21–37.

3 Fenaux P, Jouet JP, Zandecki M Lai JL, Simon M, Pollet JP, Bauters F. Chronic and subacute myelomonocytic leukaemia in the adult; a report of 60 cases with special reference to prognostic factors. *Br J Haematol* 1987; **65**: 101–106.

4 Thiede T, Engquist L, Billstrom R. Application of megakaryocytic morphology in diagnosing 5q- syndrome. *Eur J Haematol* 1988; **41**: 434–437.

5 Verhoef G, De Wolf-Peeters C, Kerim S, Van De Broeck J, Mecucci C, Van den Berghe H, Boogaerts M. Update on the prognostic implication of morphology, histology and karyotype in primary myelodysplastic syndromes. *Hematol Pathol* 1991; **5(4)**: 163–175.

6 Tricot G, De Wolf-Peeters C, Vlietinck R, Verwilghen RL. Bone marrow histology in myelodysplastic syndromes. *Br J Haematol* 1984; **58**: 217–225.

7 Kitagawa M, Kamiyama R, Takemura T, Kasuga T. Bone marrow analysis of the myelodysplastic syndromes; histological and immunohistochemical features related to the evolution of overt leukemia. *Virchows Archiv B Cell Pathol* 1989; **57**: 47–53.

8 Delacrétaz F, Schmidt P-M, Piquet D, Bachmann F, Costa J. Histopathology of myelodysplastic syndromes. *Am J Clin Pathol* 1987; **87**: 180–186.

9 Rios A, Cañizo C, Sanz MA, Vallespi T, Sanz G, Torrabadella M, Gomis F, Ruiz C, San Miguel JF. Bone marrow biopsy in myelodysplastic syndromes; morphological characteristics and contribution to study of prognostic factors. *Br J Haematol* 1990; **75**: 26–33.

10 Horny H-P, Wehrmann M, Schlicker HUH, Eichstadt A, Clemens MR, Kaiserling E. QBEND10 for the diagnosis of myelodysplastic syndromes in routinely processed bone marrow biopsy specimens. *J Clin Pathol* 1995; **48**; 291-294.

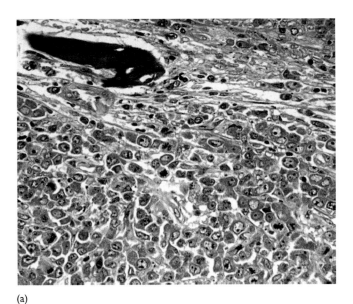

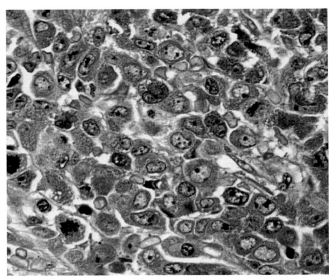

(a)

(b)

Fig 6.6 Blast crisis in CML. (a) Low power. (b) High power. Giemsa.

Histopathology of the bone marrow

The bone marrow is typically hypercellular showing profound granulocytic differentiation (Fig. 6.2).

Abnormal proliferation in the erythroid and megakaryocytic series is also frequently present although this may be minimal and require careful inspection to detect. The erythroid changes are usually those of immaturity (left-shifting). Megakaryocytes are smaller than normal, increased in number and usually mononuclear (Fig. 6.3).

Cytological atypia with clustering may be seen but is less marked than in other forms of MPD. The presence of abnormal forms around ectatic sinuses can be helpful in diagnosis, though this is more prominent as a feature of essential thrombocythaemia.

Macrophages with crystalloid inclusions ('pseudo-Gaucher' cells) (Fig. 6.4) are reported in a significant number of cases. Mast cells, plasma cells and lymphoid cells may also be present in increased numbers as a reactive phenomenon.

An increase in reticulin staining is common, with the presence of severe diffuse reticulin fibrosis being associated with a shorter survival (Fig. 6.5).

Diagnostic problems

Two situations present particular diagnostic difficulties.

1 CML VS. REACTIVE HYPERPLASIA (LEUKAEMOID REACTION)

Distinguishing between CML and a highly reactive marrow with an associated leukaemoid reaction can be difficult. Causes of such a reaction include infections, cancer outside the marrow, lymphomas and autoimmune disease. Examination for the features shown in Table 6.1 may help in making this distinction.

2 PREDICTION OF IMPENDING BLAST CRISIS, I.E. TRANSFORMATION TO ACUTE LEUKAEMIA

CML is a relentless disease progressing towards acute leukaemia, usually myeloid. The point of impending transformation cannot be detected by examination of peripheral blood or marrow smears. In the trephine it has been reported that infiltrates of blast cells and promyelocytes 4 to 8 cells thick in a perivascular and paratrabecular distribution indicates a high probability of transformation to acute leukaemia in the ensuing six months (Fig. 6.6).[3]

It has also been suggested that increased numbers of CD34 positive cells are predictive of a poorer prognosis.[4]

Polycythaemia rubra vera (PRV)
Introduction

PRV is a neoplastic proliferation with erythroid differentiation resulting in an increased mass of red blood cells. Being a myeloproliferative condition other cell lines are also involved so that an associated increase in granulocytes and platelets is common. Most cases of PRV will progress to myelofibrosis (particularly those showing marked megakaryocytic features) with subsequent blast transformation into AML.

The nomenclature of this condition varies and includes polycythaemia vera and primary proliferative polycythaemia.

Clinical features

The clinical presentation is variable and relates mainly to the patient's polycythaemia. Symptoms include headache, dizziness and visual disturbances and may be associated with gout, pruritus or occlusive vascular disease.

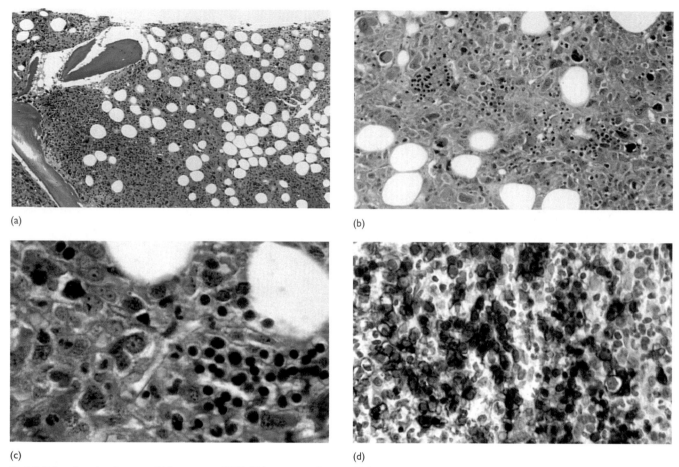

(a)

(b)

(c)

(d)

Fig 6.7 Polycythaemia rubra vera. (a) Low power. H&E. (b) Low power. Giemsa. (c) Erythroid differentiation. Giemsa. (d) Confirmed by immunostaining for glycophorin C.

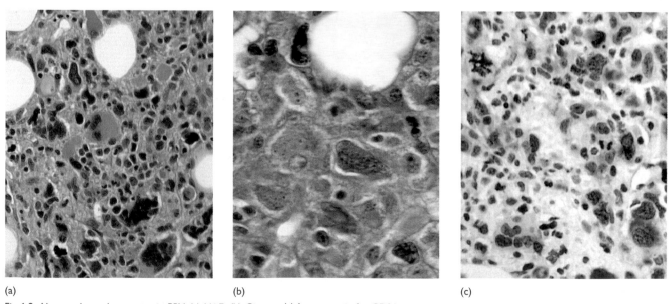

(a)

(b)

(c)

Fig 6.8 Abnormal megakaryocytes in PRV. (a) H&E. (b) Giemsa. (c) Immunostain for CD31.

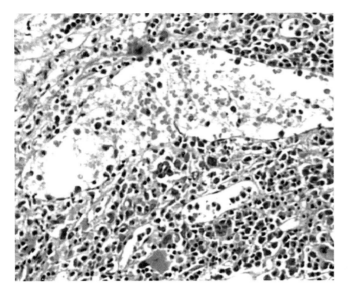

Fig 6.9 Large dilated sinus in PRV. H&E.

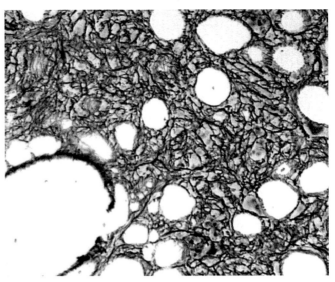

Fig 6.10 Increased reticulin in PRV.

Table 6.2 Histological features of PRV not found in CML.

Erythroid hyperplasia and paratrabecular erythroid islands
No stainable iron (metabolized by the proliferating erythroid cells)
Left-shifted granulopoiesis
Giant megakaryocytes

Histopathology of the bone marrow

The bone marrow is hypercellular with prominent erythroid differentiation (Fig. 6.7).

Florid megakaryocytic proliferation is usually present, many of which are large pleomorphic types often gathered together in prominent clusters (Fig. 6.8).

Large dilated sinuses filled with red blood cells are common (Fig. 6.9) and are usually associated with increased reticulin throughout the marrow (Fig. 6.10). Reactive plasma cells, macrophages and lymphoid cells (forming nodular aggregates in some cases) are common.

Diagnostic problems

1 DISTINCTION BETWEEN PRV AND CML WITH PROMINENT MEGAKARYOCYTES

Although these conditions are usually distinguished on clinical grounds there are a number of histological features which separate them (Table 6.2).

2 DISTINCTION BETWEEN PRV AND SECONDARY POLYCYTHAEMIA

Cytological atypia and abnormal architectural changes are absent in secondary polycythaemia. Furthermore, marrow cellularity of more than 75% and loss of the first fat space, makes a diagnosis of secondary polycythaemia unlikely.

Essential thrombocythaemia (ET)

Introduction

In this subgroup of MPD, megakaryocytes are the dominant cell line. They produce large numbers of platelets, which are often functionally impaired.

Clinical features

The disease tends to follow an indolent clinical course, but can transform into acute leukaemia. The major clinical features are illustrated in Fig. 6.11.

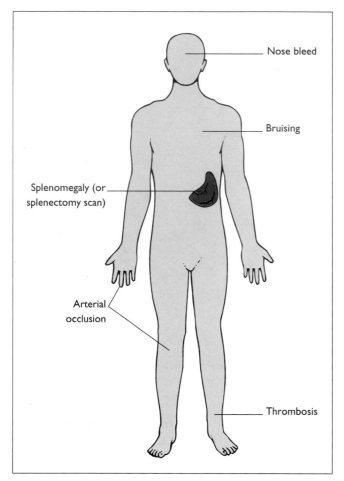

Fig 6.11 Major clinical features of essential thrombocythaemia.

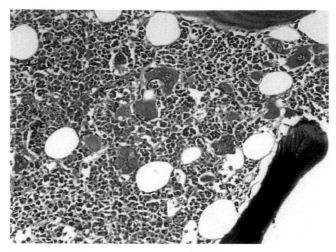

Fig 6.12 Typical low power appearance of ET. Giemsa.

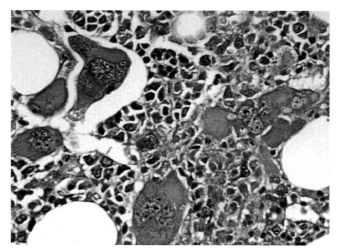

Fig 6.13 Abnormal megakaryocytes in ET. Giemsa.

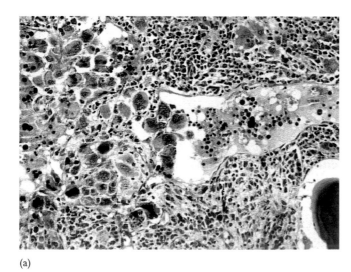

(a)

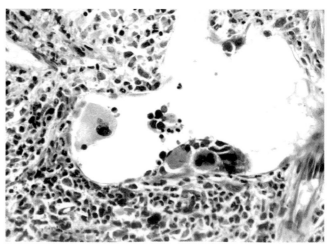

(b)

Fig 6.14 Megakaryocytes clustering around dilated sinuses. Giemsa.

Table 6.3 Causes of megakaryocytic hyperplasia.

| Post splenectomy |
| Haemorrhage |
| Malignancy |
| Crohn's disease |
| Rheumatoid arthritis |
| Hepatitis |
| Iron deficiency |

Table 6.4 Distinction between ET and reactive thrombocytosis.

ET	Reactive thrombocytosis
Megakaryocytes:	Megakaryocytes:
Giant forms	Normal or small
Clustered	Separate
Paratrabecular	Central
Atypical forms	No atypia
Emperipolesis — occasional	Emperipolesis — common
Erythropoiesis and granulopoiesis are normal	Erythropoiesis and granulopoiesis are right-shifted

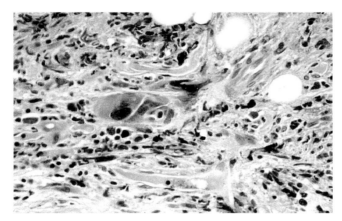

Fig 6.15 Fibrosis associated with abnormal megakaryocytes in ET. Giemsa.

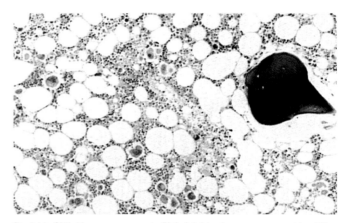

Fig 6.16 CML-like appearances in Philadelphia chromosome positive ET.

Histopathology of the bone marrow

The marrow is usually markedly hypercellular (Fig. 6.12). The hallmark is the presence of increased numbers of megakaryocytes. Many are giant forms with marked nuclear atypia (Fig. 6.13). They occur in clusters and often congregate near sinuses into which they disgorge clouds of platelets (Fig. 6.14).

Granulopoiesis and erythropoiesis are usually normal. Fibrosis is usually absent but when it occurs is considered a bad prognostic indicator. This fibrosis reflects increasing dysfunction of the megakaryocytes. This leads to local accumulation of fibrogenic platelet-derived growth factors which would normally be discharged into the circulation (Fig. 6.15).

Diagnostic problems

1 PHILADELPHIA CHROMOSOME POSITIVE CASES

Less than 10% of patients with the clinical features of ET have a Philadelphia chromosome. In these patients the marrow histology is more akin to CML (Fig. 6.16). These patients have a worse prognosis transforming to acute leukaemia in 4–7 years.[5] It is important to consider this possibility in cases of ET with atypical marrow histology.

2 ET VS. REACTIVE THROMBOCYTOSIS

Certain conditions can produce large numbers of megakaryocytes in the bone marrow. A brief list is given in Table 6.3. If fibrosis is also present one should look for evidence of metastatic carcinoma in the marrow since this can produce megakaryocytic hyperplasia which might be misdiagnosed as MPD (Table 6.4).

Primary myelofibrosis
Chronic myelofibrosis

This is probably not a separate entity but represents a response by the marrow to the presence of the neoplastic cells in one of the other forms of MPD. The fibrosis results from fibroblast stimulation by platelet-derived growth factors released by dysfunctional megakaryocytes (Fig. 6.15).

When the fibrosis occurs as the dominant feature in the marrow at presentation it is referred to as chronic primary myelofibrosis. It may then not be possible to identify the abnormalities of a pre-existing subgroup of MPD. PRV, ET and CML can all evolve into myelofibrosis. When this progression is clearly documented this is known as secondary myelofibrosis. In practice these conditions are often indistinguishable.

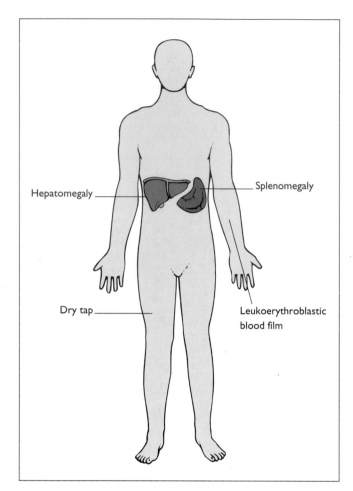

Hepatomegaly

Splenomegaly

Dry tap

Leukoerythroblastic blood film

Fig 6.17 MPD – myelofibrosis.

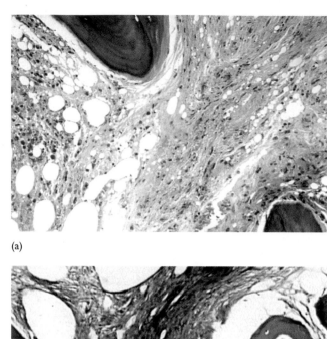

(a)

(b)

Fig 6.18 Dense fibrosis in primary myelofibrosis. (a) Giemsa. (b) Reticulin.

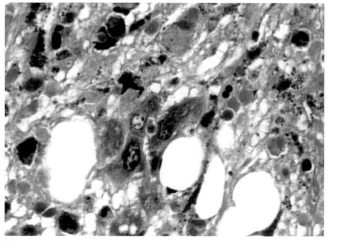

(a)

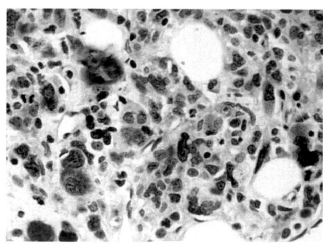

(b)

Fig 6.19 Abnormal megakaryocytic myelofibrosis. (a) Giemsa. (b) Immunostain for CD31.

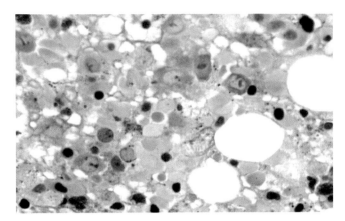

Fig 6.20 PRV-like area in primary myelofibrosis. Giemsa.

Clinical features
These are summarized in Fig. 6.17.

Histopathology of the bone marrow
The morphology is characterized by well-vascularized fibrosis radiating from endosteal and pericapillary regions (Fig. 6.18). In some

cases there is osteoblastic proliferation with new bone formation, often referred to as osteomyelofibrosis. It is nearly always possible to identify abnormal megakaryocytes within this fibrosis although immunostaining may be necessary to confirm their lineage (Fig. 6.19). A thorough search of a myelofibrotic trephine will usually reveal areas of underlying MPD (Fig. 6.20) although it is believed that some cases are entirely primary (also known as agnogenic myelofibrosis).

ACUTE MYELOFIBROSIS
There are two acute fibrotic conditions which have been referred to under this name. The commoner is probably acute megakaryoblastic (M7) leukaemia without blast cells in the peripheral blood. In the other, which is rare, this relationship is arguable. Here the picture is dominated by pancytopenia and a rapid downhill course without any real evidence of leukaemia. The marrow histology is hypocellular with the fat spaces replaced by highly vascular fibrous tissue (Fig. 6.21).[6]

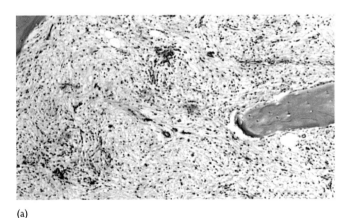
(a)

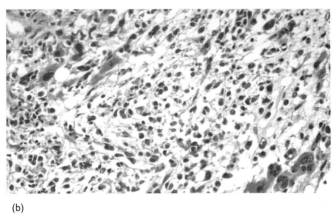
(b)

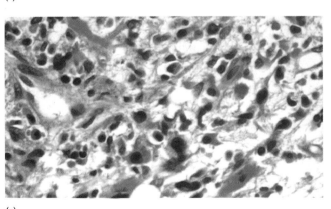
(c)

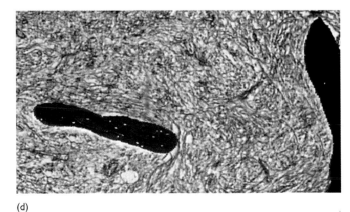
(d)

Fig 6.21 Acute myelofibrosis (of M7 type). (a – c) H&E. (d) Reticulin.

Table 6.5. Causes of secondary diffuse fibrosis in the bone marrow.

All other myeloproliferations
Acute leukaemias other than M7
MDS
Lymphoma: both Hodgkin's and non-Hodgkin's
Myeloma
Carcinoma and sarcoma
TB and other granulomatous disorders
Others including fractures, toxins and irradiation

Table 6.6 Comparison of MDS with MPD.

MDS	MPD
Abnormal topography	Normal topography
Immaturity	Usually full maturity
Ineffective haematopoiesis, i.e. 'paenias'	Effective haematopoiesis, i.e. 'cytosis'
Stem cell defect reflected as premalignant, i.e. dysplastic changes	Stem cell defect reflected as frankly malignant changes

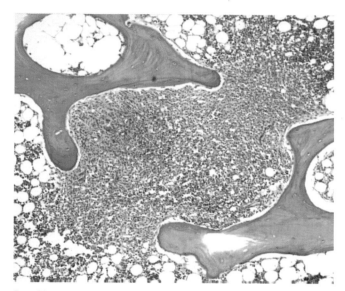

Fig 6.22 Hypercellular bone marrow in mastocytosis. H&E.

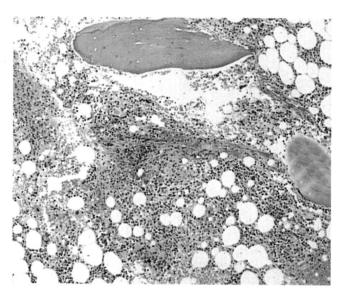

Fig 6.23 (a)

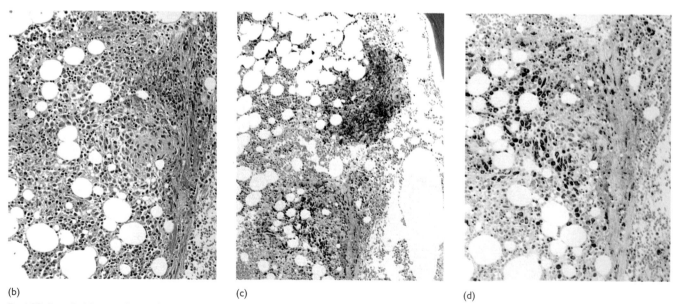

(b)　　　　　(c)　　　　　(d)

Fig 6.23 So-called 'mast cell granulomas' in systemic mastocytosis. (a & b) H&E. (c & d) Giemsa.

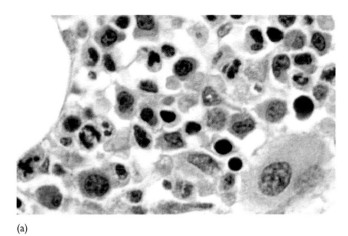

(a)

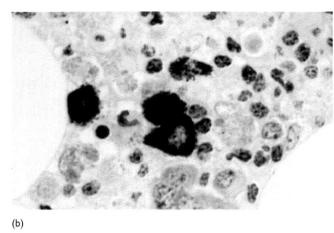

(b)

Fig 6.24 Cytological appearances of mastocytosis. (a) H&E. (b) Giemsa.

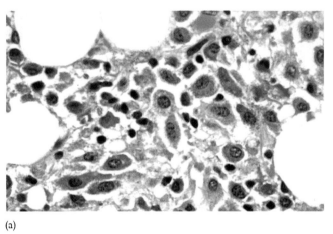

(a)

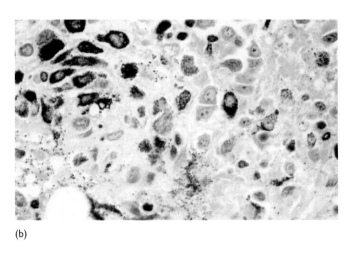

(b)

Fig 6.25 Granulation in mast cells. (a) H&E. (b) Giemsa.

Diagnostic difficulties

DISTINCTION FROM OTHER FORMS OF FIBROSIS

A number of other conditions may cause extensive marrow fibrosis and should be considered in the differential diagnosis (Table 6.5).

DISTINGUISHING BETWEEN MDS AND MPD (Table 6.6)

There is no doubt that a number of patients seem to show features, both clinically and histologically, of MDS and MPD. This may reflect imprecision in the current means of classifying these disorders although it is more likely that biologically there is considerable overlap between them. Karyotype analysis is becoming increasingly important in providing more objective criteria.

Mast cell disease

Neoplastic conditions of mast cells are rare.[7,8] This has resulted in a lack of reliable information on the clinical course and histological classification. The only entity likely to be encountered in the bone marrow is systemic mastocytosis (SM). This has two forms:

1 BENIGN

This is associated with skin involvement (urticaria pigmentosa) and is rarely associated with myeloproliferative disorders.

2 MALIGNANT

This is not associated with urticaria pigmentosa. However, 75% of cases will be associated with MPD with some progress to acute leukaemia. Mast cell leukaemia is rare.

Histopathology of the bone marrow

The marrow is usually hypercellular (Fig. 6.22) and focally infiltrated by aggregates of mast cells often known as mast cell granulomas. These may have a perivascular and paratrabecular distribution (Fig. 6.23). The infiltrate consists of mast cells, lymphocytes, plasma cells, eosinophils and sea-green histiocytes (Fig. 6.24) surrounding the mast cell precursors in the granulomas. These cells have a bland cytological appearance, they may be spindled and their nuclei are round or oval and may be indented. The granules may be apparent on H&E but are better appreciated on Giemsa (Fig. 6.25), toluidine blue or naphthol-AS-D-chloracetate esterase (Leder) stains.

The infiltrate is often associated with fibrosis, an increased number of eosinophils and bone changes which may include osteosclerosis, osteopaenia and osteolysis. Some patients have widespread osteoporosis. Distinguishing between the benign and malignant forms histologically is not always possible. In benign SM the mast cells do not show cytological atypia, the marrow fat is preserved and the infiltrate is nodular rather than diffuse. This contrasts with the malignant form of SM where the amount of marrow fat is reduced and the mast cells may be atypical, diffusely infiltrative and are likely to be accompanied by the histological features of MPD.

A very uncommon mast cell proliferation known as 'eosinophilic histiocytic lesion' appears to involve only the bone marrow and can be histologically indistinguishable from SM.[9]

Differential diagnosis

The focal pattern of involvement which often occurs in SM may superficially resemble that of Hodgkin's disease of the marrow where focal areas of fibrosis are seen. In addition, both entities may contain considerable numbers of eosinophils. However, the presence of large atypical cells with prominent eosinophilic nucleoli, i.e. Hodgkin and Reed–Sternberg cells and/or the appropriate immunocytochemistry, will exclude SM (Table 6.7).

Although most anti-CD68s will show some positivity it is useful to employ those antibodies, e.g. KP1, recognizing the granulocytic end of the spectrum for stronger, more robust staining of this condition (Fig. 6.26).

Reactive marrows in HIV-positive patients occasionally show aggregates of fibroblasts, lymphocytes and macrophages, raising a possibility of mast cell disease. Special stains for mast cell granules will be negative.

Table 6.7 Immunocytochemical distinction of systemic mastocytosis (SM) and Hodgkin's disease (HD).

Antigen	SM	HD
CD30	–	+
CD68	+	–

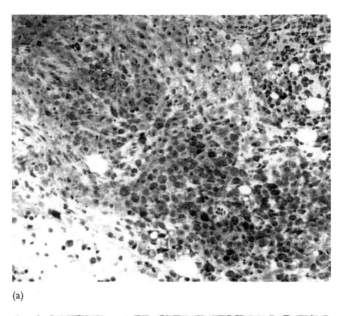

(a)

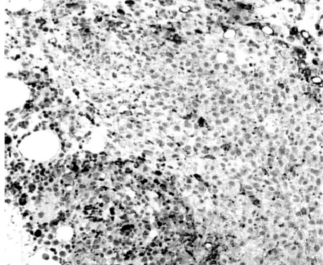

(b)

Fig 6.26 Typical immunostaining of systematic mastocytosis for CD68. Note that the degree of staining varies with the antibody chosen, e.g. (a) KP1 diffuse cytoplasmic, (b) PGM1 dot-like cytoplasmic.

References

1 Frisch B, Bartl R, Jaeger K. Histological diagnosis of chronic myeloproliferative disorders (CMPD). *Hematol Rev* 1989; **3**; 131–147.

2 Martiat P, Michaux JL, Rodhain. Philadelphia-negative (Ph-) Chronic myeloid leukaemia (CML): comparison with Ph+ CML and Chronic myelomonocytic leukaemia. *Blood* 1991; **78**: 205–211.

3 Islam A. Prediction of impending blast cell transformation in chronic-granulocytic leukaemia. *Histopathology* 1988; **12**: 633–639.

4 Orazi A, Neiman R, Cauling H, Heerme N, John K. CD34 Immunostaining of bone marrow biopsy specimens is a reliable way to classify the phases of chronic myeloid leukaemia. *Am J Clin Pathol* 1994; **101**: 426–428.

5 Stoll DB, Peterson P, Exten R, Laslo J, Pisciotta AV, Ellis JT, White P, Vaidya K, Bozdech M, Murphy S. Clinical presentation and natural history of patients with esssential thrombocythemia and the Philadelphia chromosome. *Am J Hematol* 1991; **27**: 87–97.

6 Hruban RH, Kuhajda FP, Mann RB. Acute myelofibrosis. Immunohistochemical study of four cases and comparison with acute megakaryocytic leukaemia. *Am J Clin Pathol* 1987; **88**: 578–588.

7 Horny H-P, Parwaresch MR, Lennert K. Bone marrow findings in systemic mastocytosis. *Hum Pathol* 1985; **16**: 808–814.

8 Lennert K, Parwaresch MR. Mast cells and mast cell neoplasia: a review. *Histopathology* 1979; **3**: 349–365.

9 Rywlin AM, Hoffman EP, Ortega RS. Eosinophilic fibrohistiocytic lesion of bone marrow. A distinctive new morphological finding, probably related to drug hypersensitivity. *Blood* 1972; **40**: 464–472.

Acute leukaemia

Chapter 7

Introduction

There are two main types of acute leukaemia, myeloid (AML) and lymphoblastic (ALL). Acute leukaemias are blastic proliferations of white cells which usually but not invariably involve the peripheral blood. The exact definition of particular subtypes is often arbitrary (defined by committee consensus) and much unnecessary confusion between histologist and haematologist/oncologist can be avoided by comparing specimens and relating findings to individual patients. This is especially the case when dealing with the overlap between lymphoma and leukaemia.

Both acute leukaemias affect all ages although their frequencies are quite different. AML is primarily an adult disease with the incidence rising with age whereas more than 85% of cases of ALL are in children aged under 15. The prognosis in ALL in children is excellent whereas in AML it is generally poor, particularly in the elderly. Some studies give those over 55 years old only a 2% chance of 5-year survival regardless of therapy.

Classification

The French, American and British (FAB) group classification has been widely accepted especially for both AML and ALL.[1,2] This classification is based on cytological appearances that are not always best appreciated in trephine sections. Appropriate immunostaining and liaison with the Haematology Department considerably aid an accurate diagnosis.

Acute myeloid leukaemia (AML)
Classification

For the examination of trephine sections the FAB classification can be summarized in Table 7.1.

Histopathology and immunophenotyping

ACUTE MYELOID LEUKAEMIA M0–M5

It may seem almost sacreligious to state, but with the exception of acute promyelocytic leukaemia (bi-lobed nuclei, cytoplasmic granules) the first five categories of the FAB classification look remarkably similar on histology. Worse still there are at present no reliable antibodies functioning on fixed sections to aid in their positive identification. An exception is that most cases of M4 and M5 show dot-like cytoplasmic labelling for CD68. Staining of myeloperoxidase or elastase is helpful but cannot always be demonstrated although advances such as antigen retrieval have made significant improvements.

FAB category	Criteria	Other name(s)
M0	No differentiation	AML
M1	Myeloid without maturation	AML
M2	Myeloid with maturation	AML
M3	Bilobed hypergranulated blasts	Acute promyelocytic leukaemia (APML)
M4	Mixed granulocytic/monocytic differentiation	Acute myelomonocytic leukaemia (AMML)
M5	Monocytic/blastic	Acute monocytic leukaemia (AMoL)
M6	Erythroid	Acute erythroleukaemia
M7	Megakaryocytic/blastic	Acute megakaryocytic leukaemia

Table 7.1 FAB classification for the examination of bone marrow trephines.

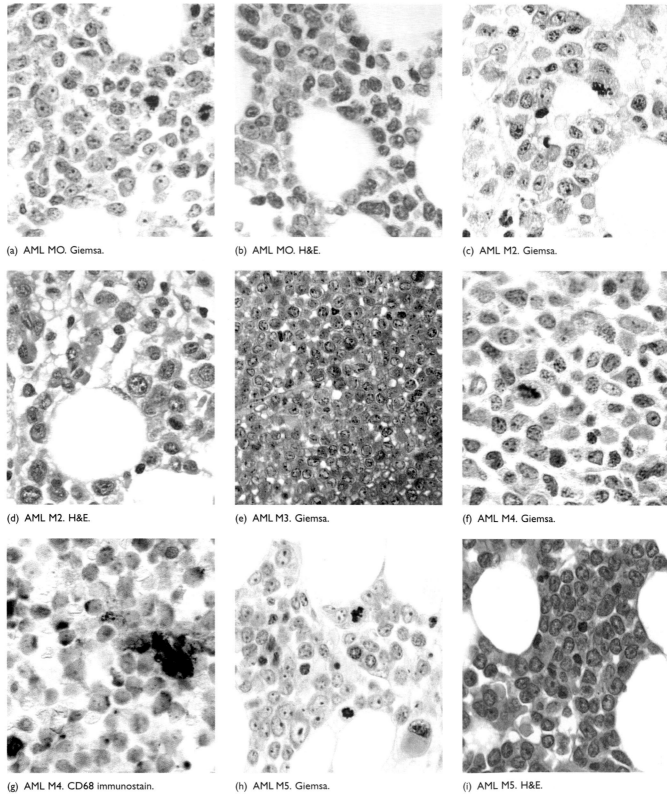

(a) AML MO. Giemsa.

(b) AML MO. H&E.

(c) AML M2. Giemsa.

(d) AML M2. H&E.

(e) AML M3. Giemsa.

(f) AML M4. Giemsa.

(g) AML M4. CD68 immunostain.

(h) AML M5. Giemsa.

(i) AML M5. H&E.

Fig 7.1 Typical histological picture of trephines from the different AML FAB categories.

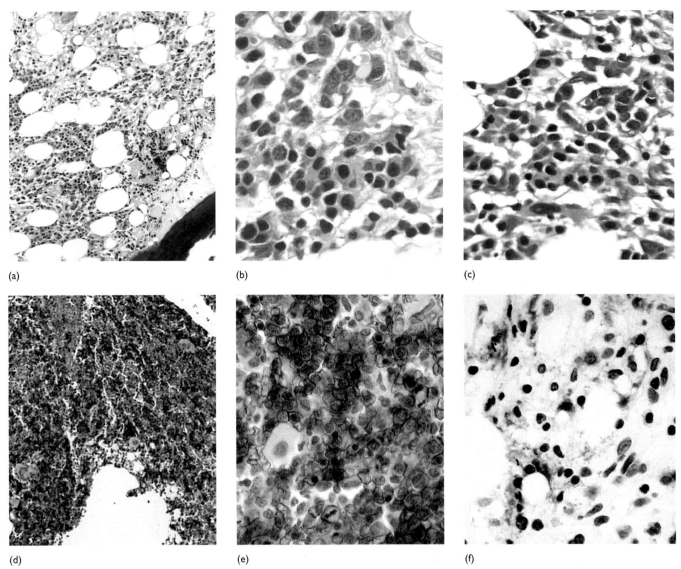

(a)   (b)   (c)

(d)   (e)   (f)

Fig 7.2 M6 erythroleukaemia. The histology is shown in (a) & (b) Giemsa and (c) H&E. The majority of the cells are erythroid as shown by glycophorin C staining (d) & (e) but many abnormal cells express other lineage markers such as the megakaryocytic antigen CD61 (f).

Examples of the trephine histology of each category from M0 to M5 (apart from M1) are given below and it can be seen that without careful liaison with the Haematology Department it would be difficult to distinguish these (Fig. 7.1).

ERYTHROLEUKAEMIA M6

This is a rare category which it is easy to overlook as myelodysplasia with excess blasts. The erythroid element is predominantly associated with dysplastic erythroid colonies whereas the lineage of most of the true leukaemic blasts is uncertain (Fig. 7.2).

MEGAKARYOBLASTIC AND MEGAKARYOCYTIC LEUKAEMIA M7

This acute leukaemia has a variable morphology from the recognizably megakaryocytic to the frankly bizarre where it can be identified only on the basis of immunocytochemistry. As mentioned in Chapter 6 on myeloproliferative diseases, most cases of acute myelofibrosis are examples of M7 leukaemia (Fig. 7.3).

HYPOPLASTIC AML

These patients present with pancytopaenia and a 'dry tap' at aspiration. Aplastic anaemia is usually the main differential, though leukaemia is often suspected clinically due to a few suspicious blast-like cells being seen in the peripheral blood. The trephine usually

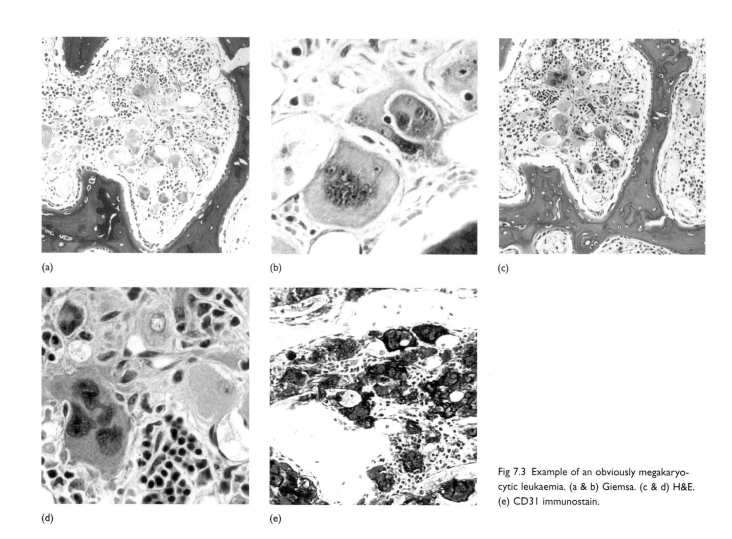

(a)

(b)

(c)

(d)

(e)

Fig 7.3 Example of an obviously megakaryo-cytic leukaemia. (a & b) Giemsa. (c & d) H&E. (e) CD31 immunostain.

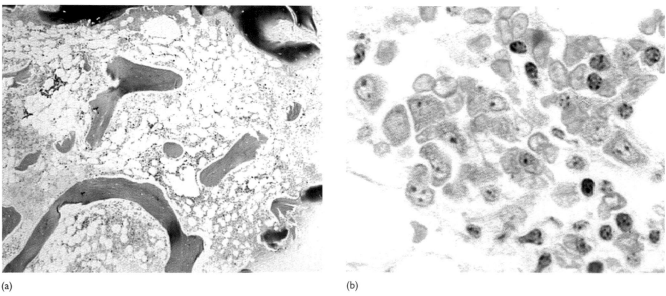

(a)

(b)

Fig 7.4 An example of a hypocellular marrow (a) in which the majority of cells present are clearly blasts. (b) Giemsa.

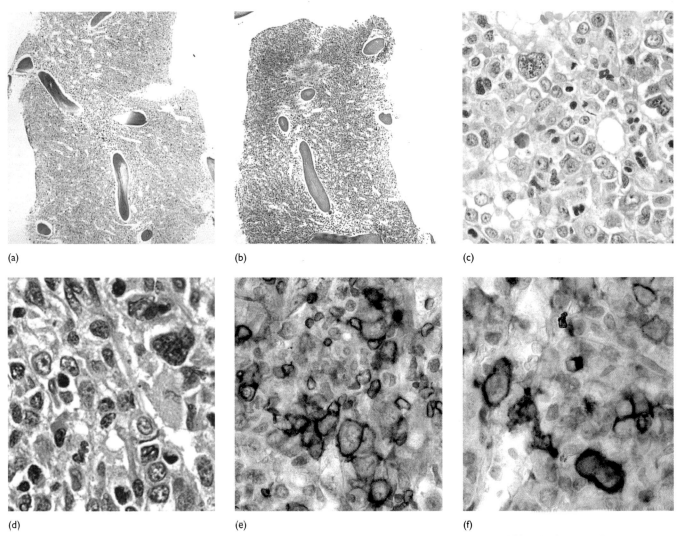

Fig 7.5 Hypercellular marrow (a & b) packed with abnormal pleomorphic blasts (c & d), some expressing erythroid (e) and others megakaryocytic (f) antigens. (a & c) Giemsa. (b & d) H&E. (e & f) Immunoperoxidase.

makes the diagnosis by showing discrete collections of primitive blast cells in an otherwise empty marrow. It is said that hypocellular AML should be distinguished from hypocellular MDS. It is common to find evidence of both conditions so that distinguishing hypocellular AML from refractory anaemia with excess blasts is not always easy. AML should not be diagnosed unless more than 30% of the cells can be clearly identified as blast cells (Fig. 7.4).

Diagnostic problems

UNCLASSIFIABLE CASES

Leukaemia is no different to most other tumour classifications with cases showing overlapping features. In the case of AML the histologist will probably not become involved in disputes over M0 to M5 but occasional bizarre cases spanning M6 and M7 do occur (Fig. 7.5).

AML OR ALL

It is frequently difficult to decide on histological grounds whether an acute leukaemia is lymphoid or myeloid. Antibodies against the B cell antigen CD79a have now come to the rescue since this antigen is expressed on virtually all cases of ALL, except of course for the rare T cell cases where antibodies to a number of T cell antigens may be used instead (Fig. 7.6).

In these cases the pathologist needs to be cautious not to overlook those biphenotypic leukaemias which express both lymphoid and myeloid markers. Unfortunately until a suitable myeloid panel of antibodies becomes available for trephine sections we will have to rely on liaison with the Haematology Department to make this diagnosis.

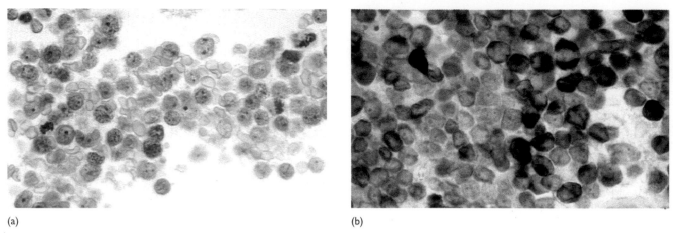

(a)   (b)

Fig 7.6 Case of ALL initially believed to be AML on cytological and histological grounds. (a) Giemsa. It was negative for all myeloid markers but expressed CD79a, a B cell antigen (b), as well as other ALL markers such as CD10.

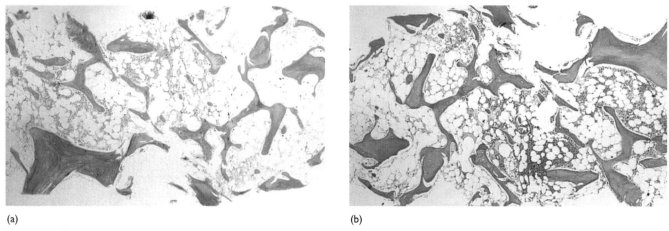

(a)   (b)

Fig 7.7 Typical empty marrow seen a week or so after transplantation. (a) Giemsa. (b) H&E.

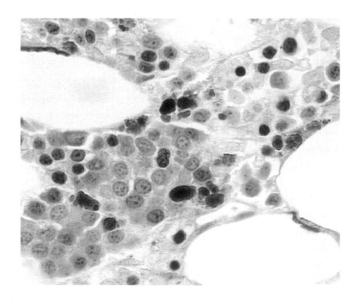

Fig 7.8 Regenerating erythroid colonies about one month after engraftment.

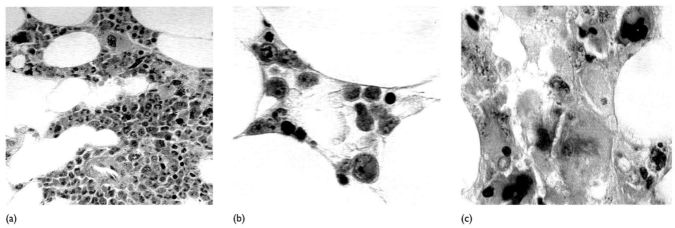

(a)   (b)   (c)

Fig 7.9 Relatively normal cellularity a few months after engraftment. (a) Giemsa, but note the dysplastic erythroid cells. (b) Giemsa and megakaryocytes. (c) Giemsa, which should not be confused with leukaemic relapse.

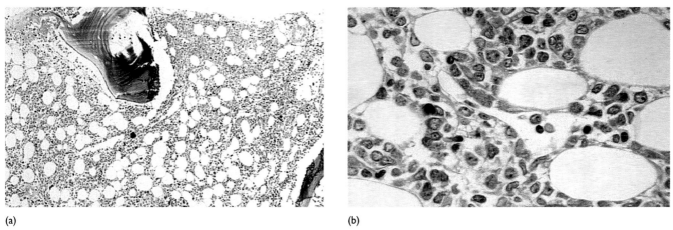

(a)   (b)

Fig 7.10 Leukaemic relapse six years after a successful engraftment for AML. Note that the marrow is full of primitive blast cells. (a) Low power. (b) High power. Both Giemsa.

Acute lymphoblastic leukaemia (ALL)

Reflecting the histological bias of the authors, a full presentation of this topic will be found in the chapter on lymphoma.

Transplantation and graft-versus-host disease

The place of bone marrow transplantation in the treatment of both haematological and other malignancies is still not fully established. Many, if not most procedures, remain experimental, so close liaison with appropriate clinicians is essential in the interpretation of bone marrow and other histology from these patients. Three approaches are currently in use employing allografts, autografts and peripheral stem cell rescue. All of these employ prior intensive chemotherapy so that initial bone marrow samples are characterized by severe hypocellularity (Fig. 7.7).

The marrow regeneration is usually led by erythropoiesis followed by megakaryocytic and granulocytic proliferation (Fig. 7.8).

Without too many complications the marrow regenerates steadily to produce relatively normal indices in the peripheral blood over a period of a few months. During this period the regenerating colonies can appear profoundly dysplastic which should not be misinterpreted as a recurrence of tumour (Fig. 7.9).

Relapse of a leukaemia or lymphoma may occur at any time even after several years and is typically dramatic (Fig. 7.10).

An early complication is failed or slow regeneration. These are being treated with a number of recombinant growth factors which themselves can produce dysplastic or bizarre appearances. Infectious complications are unfortunately common and include viral, fungal and mycobacterial diseases whose appearances are the same as those seen in other immunocompromised individuals.

The haematopathologist is often asked to diagnose acute graft-versus-host disease in skin or rectal biopsies of allograft patients. When severe the diagnosis is clinically obvious but mild cases are

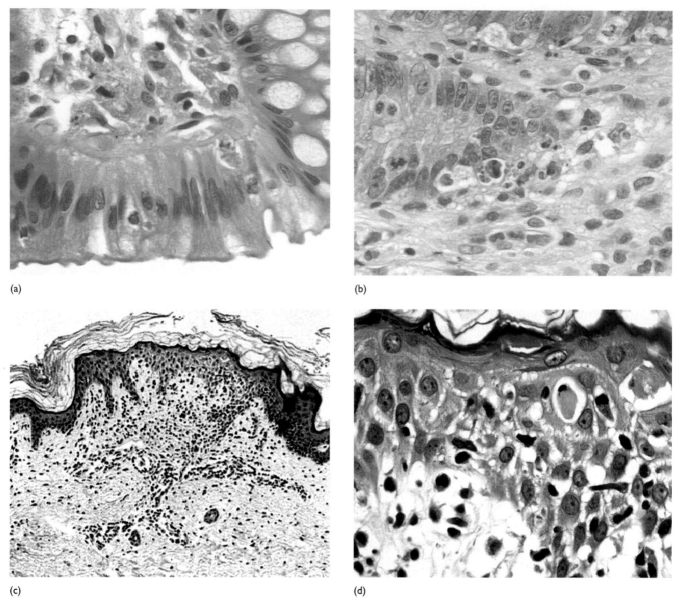

(a)

(b)

(c)

(d)

Fig 7.11 Typical graft-versus-host disease in a bone marrow allograft recipient. (a & b) Show mild and severe involvement of rectal mucosa and (c & d) illustrate severe skin disease at low and high power.

indistinguishable from drug-induced changes and only careful clinical review can separate these. There is now a growing consensus that mild graft-versus-host disease in allografted patients is beneficial due to an associated graft versus leukaemia or lymphoma reaction (Fig. 7.11).

References

1 Bennett JM, Catovsky D, Daniel MT, *et al*. Proposals for the classification of the acute leukaemias (FAB cooperative group). *Br J Haematol* 1976; **33**: 451–458.

2 Bennett JM, Catovsky D, Daniel MT, *et al*. Proposed revised criteria for the classification of acute myeloid leukaemia. *Ann Intern Med* 1985; **103**: 626–629.

Lymphomas

Introduction

There can be few areas of histopathology encountered by the general surgical pathologist which produce such a 'heart sink' feeling as lymphoma classification. The apparent difficulty with lymphoma classification has been partly due to the genuine complexity of the subject with the constant need to update classifications in the light of scientific advances and partly because of the existence of a number of influential pathologists, many with strong personalities, who have actively promoted their own classifications in an atmosphere which was more competitive than co-operative.

The historical perspective outlining the development of lymphoma classification is shown in Table 8.1. No classification exists which is perfect but in the final analysis the purpose of a classification is to provide clinically relevant information in terms of prognosis and predicting behaviour and in determining the most effective therapeutic regimes. It should be understandable, reproducible and based on concepts which have scientific credibility.

What does the clinician require from the pathologist?

The clinician will need to know the following so that the appropriate therapy can be given:
(a) is it Hodgkin's or non-Hodgkin's disease?
(b) if it is Hodgkin's disease, which subtype?
(c) if it is non-Hodgkin's disease, what is the subtype and is it likely to be high-grade or low-grade?
(d) is there histological evidence of marrow involvement?
The following chapters discuss a variety of lymphomas selected from the REAL classification (which has been incorporated as the latest WHO classification of lymphomas) and they are presented largely in that format. We regard them as representing the lymphomas most likely to be encountered by the general surgical pathologist. Some of the more frequently encountered entities will be described in greater detail.

Those lymphomas to be discussed are:

Non-Hodgkin's Lymphoma

B cell	Lymphoblastic
	Lymphocytic
	Lymphoplasmacytic/Immunocytoma
	Mantle cell
	Follicular
	Marginal zone
	Hairy cell
	Multiple myeloma
	Large cell
	Burkitt's

T cell	Lymphoblastic
	Lymphocytic
	Primary cutaneous, i.e. MF/SS
	Large granular lymphocyte
	Peripheral, *unspecified*
	which includes the following
	categories of the Kiel classification:
	• Lennert's
	• Pleomorphic
	• T-zone
	Angioimmunoblastic
	Adult T cell
	Anaplastic large cell

Hodgkin's disease	Classical subtypes
	• nodular sclerosis
	• mixed cellularity
	Lymphocyte predominance

Table 8.1 Historical perspective of the development of lymphoma classification.

1870s Concept of malignant lymphoma originated by Billroth.

1890s Recognition of Hodgkin's and non-Hodgkin's lymphomas as separate disease groups by Dreschfeld and Kundrat.

1900-1950 Awareness of different groups within the non-Hodgkin's lymphomas but the terminology used was not standardized and certain terms meant different things to different pathologists, e.g. lymphosarcoma, reticulum cell sarcoma.

1960s Emergence of the first clinically useful classifications in terms of providing prognostic information. These were the Rappaport classification for non-Hodgkin's lymphoma and the Lukes-Butler classification for Hodgkin's disease. Rappaport classified lymphomas primarily on the growth pattern, i.e. nodular or diffuse and also placed some weight on the degree of differentiation and morphological similarity of the malignant cell compared to either normal small lymphocytes or histiocytes (hence the erroneous term 'histiocytic lymphoma'; these lymphoma cells are now known to be transformed lymphocytes).

1970s Increasing knowledge of the functional and morphological heterogeneity of the immune system, e.g. T and B cells led to modification of Rappaport's classification to recognize additional specific entities, e.g. Burkitt's and lymphoblastic lymphoma.

1975 Increased recognition by haematopathologists of the large number of morphologically different lymphoid cells within normal lymphoid tissue led to classifications based on detailed morphological descriptions of lymphoid cells. The front-runners of this type of classification were, in Europe, Professor Lennert's Kiel classification and, in the United States, the Lukes/Collins classification. Both attempted to postulate an origin for various lymphomas from normal cells within lymph nodes, e.g. follicular lymphoma cells had their normal counterpart in germinal centres of secondary lymphoid follicles. Around the same time a number of others produced similar classifications also largely based on the appearance of the malignant cells.

1980s The large number of classifications at this time created a lot of confusion and frustration amongst clinicians and physicians. This prompted the National Cancer Institute to facilitate the development of a *Working formulation for clinical usage*. This was to serve as a 'Rosetta stone' for lymphoma classifications allowing translation of one classification's terminology into another's. Although it was not intended as a classification it became one for many pathologists and clinicians, particularly in the USA.

1990 The Kiel classification was updated to take account of advances in immunology and molecular genetics; it included a classification of T cell lymphomas. The major emphasis was still on the morphological detail of the lymphoma cells as revealed by the Giemsa stain. The preference in the USA and the UK for haematoxylin and eosin stain partly limited the use of this classification in these countries. Many felt that the subtle nuances in cytological detail described by Lennert were beyond the average jobbing surgical pathologist. As one delegate declared during debate at an international lymphoma meeting 'we don't all have Lennert's eyes'.

1995 The Revised European and American Lymphoma (REAL) classification was proposed by the 19 members of the International Lymphoma Study Group as a consensus classification which draws on the best of current classifications, in particular the Kiel classification, but also incorporates and emphasizes other facets in lymphoma diagnosis, e.g. immunophenotype, genetics and clinical features. In so doing, it moved away from the concept of lymphomas belonging strictly to low or high-grade groups and emphasized the heterogeneity of clinical behaviour within specific lymphoma types, e.g. not all follicular lymphomas have an indolent clinical course. Lymphomas should be viewed as having a range of possible differentiations in the same way as neoplasms of other tissues. The REAL classification, unlike others, has incorporated Hodgkin's disease and attempted to clarify the different subtypes using the same format that it applied to the non-Hodgkin's lymphomas.

The future As our knowledge of lymphomas increases, particularly at a molecular level, new classifications will be developed with more relevance to therapy and prognosis. Pathologists and clinicians must resign themselves to further change in lymphoma classification.

The Revised European American Lymphoma/World Health Organisation classification

The following is a brief overview of the consensus proposal on lymphoma classification from the International Lymphoma Study Group. This classification has been adopted as the WHO classification of lymphoma.

Precursor B cell neoplasms
Precursor B lymphoblastic leukaemia/lymphoma

Peripheral B cell neoplasms
B cell chronic lymphocytic leukaemia/prolymphocytic leukaemia/small lymphocytic lymphoma
Immunocytoma/lymphoplasmacytoid lymphoma
Mantle cell lymphoma
Follicle centre cell lymphoma, follicular
Marginal zone B cell lymphoma
Hairy cell leukaemia
Plasmacytoma/plasma cell myeloma
Diffuse large B cell lymphoma
Burkitt's lymphoma

This list excludes provisional categories

B cell neoplasms in the REAL classification

The REAL classification focuses attention on non-Hodgkin's lymphoma although, unlike previous schemes, it also covers Hodgkin's disease. Ten of the non-Hodgkin's lymphomas are of B lymphoid origin, and these are divided into those arising from immature cells, and those representing more mature B cells.

B LYMPHOBLASTIC LEUKAEMIA/LYMPHOMA

Lymphoblastic neoplasms of B cell type usually present as a leukaemia (Fig. 8.1). They typically express markers, such as terminal transferase and CD10, found on early B cells. The CD79a antigen is of value, since it is often the only B cell marker expressed by these cells which is detectable in paraffin embedded tissue.

Although bone marrow and blood involvement is very common, a few cases are localized as solid tumours, usually in lymph nodes. The disease, though aggressive, can be cured, particularly when it occurs in children.

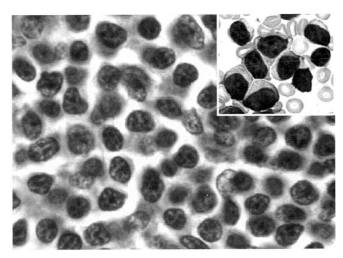

Fig 8.2 B cell small lymphocytic lymphoma.

B CELL LYMPHOCYTIC LYMPHOMA

Neoplasms composed of small lymphocytes may present as lymphomas or leukaemias (Fig. 8.2). The leukaemias comprise both chronic lymphocytic and prolymphocytic leukaemia. Histologically, small lymphocytic neoplasms show a monotonous infiltration of small cells, but clusters of larger cells ('pseudofollicles or proliferation centres') are a common feature. Occasionally the neoplastic cells may differentiate to the plasma cell stage but this should not prompt a diagnosis of immunocytoma. Small lymphocytic neoplasms usually express CD5 and CD23, in addition to 'pan-B cell' markers. They tend to follow an indolent course.

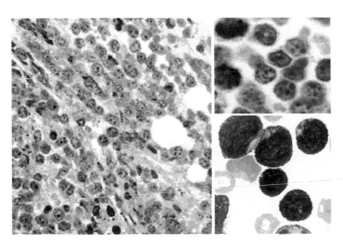

Fig 8.1 B lymphoblastic leukaemia/lymphoma.

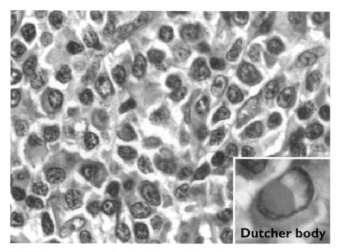

Fig 8.3 Immunocytoma/lymphoplasmacytic lymphoma.

IMMUNOCYTOMA/ LYMPHOPLASMACYTIC LYMPHOMA

The neoplastic cell in immunocytoma (also known as lympho-plasmacytic lymphoma) (Fig 8.3) is a B lymphocyte, which shows a tendency to differentiate towards the plasma cell stage. IgM is detectable in the cells with plasmacytic features, within the cyto-plasm or as intranuclear inclusions (Dutcher bodies). IgM may also appear in the serum as a paraprotein, and the disease then corre-sponds to Waldenström's macroglobulinemia. Strong cytoplasmic IgM positivity can help to distinguish the disease from small lym-phocytic neoplasms, as does the absence of CD5. The disease is normally indolent but may transform to an aggressive large cell lym-phoma. Other B cell neoplasms (e.g. small lymphocytic lymphoma and MALT lymphoma) may show plasmacytoid differentiation, and a diagnosis of immunocytoma should only be made in cases lacking features of other neoplasms.

FOLLICLE CENTRE CELL LYMPHOMA

Follicular lymphoma (Fig. 8.4) constitutes, at least in the West, one of the most frequent non-Hodgkin's lymphomas, and it is clear that they are the neoplastic equivalent of normal germinal centres. This origin explains their title in the Kiel scheme of 'centroblastic/ centrocytic' lymphoma. They are usually easy to recognize because of their follicular growth pattern. They occasionally transform into diffuse tumours containing numerous large cells (centroblasts), and then fall into the group of 'large B cell lymphoma'. The (14;18) chro-mosomal translocation, present in two thirds to three quarters of cases, juxtaposes the BCL-2 gene to the Ig heavy chain gene, and this is accompanied by expression of BCL-2 protein. This is in contrast to normal germinal centre B cells, which are BCL-2—negative. Fol-licular lymphomas that lack this translocation usually also express BCL-2 protein and show identical clinical behaviour to transloca-tion-positive cases. The disease is usually only slowly progressive but is essentially incurable.

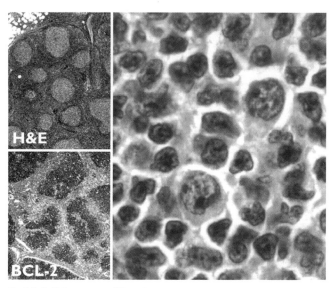

Fig 8.4 Follicle centre cell lymphoma.

MANTLE CELL LYMPHOMA

Mantle cell lymphoma (Fig. 8.5) is equivalent to 'centrocytic lym-phoma' in the Kiel scheme. This change of name reflects the lack of evidence that the neoplastic cells derive from a germinal centre cell (as the term 'centrocytic' implies), and the realization that they have many of the features of mantle zone lymphocytes.

The disease usually presents with lymphadenopathy, but may be found at extranodal sites, notably the gastrointestinal tract (lymphomatous polyposis). The neoplastic cells are usually small to medium-sized and may have irregular or 'cleaved' nuclei, or a more 'blastic' appearance. The growth pattern is often nodular and the neoplastic cells tend to 'home' to the mantle zones of lymphoid follicles.

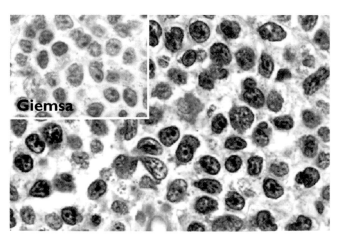

Fig 8.5 Mantle cell lymphoma.

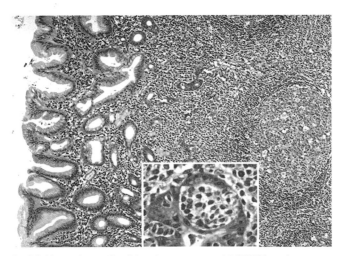

Fig 8.6 Marginal zone B cell lymphoma, extranodal (MALT-type).

HAIRY CELL LEUKAEMIA

Hairy cell leukaemia (Fig. 8.7) is characterized by cells with fine villous surface projections and bean-shaped nuclei, which are seen in the circulation, the bone marrow and the red pulp of the spleen. The latter sites of involvement account for pancytopenia and marked splenomegaly. Lymph node infiltration is rare. The cells express, in addition to typical B cell antigens, the receptor for interleukin 2 (CD25) and the CD103 integrin (a cell adhesion molecule). In paraffin sections a distinctive pattern of markers can be detected, and these may be of diagnostic value, e.g. when the marrow shows a low level of infiltration. In addition to pan-B markers such as CD20 and CD79, neoplastic cells express CD68 (as cytoplasmic dots) and are labelled by antibody DBA.44. The disease tends to follow an indolent course.

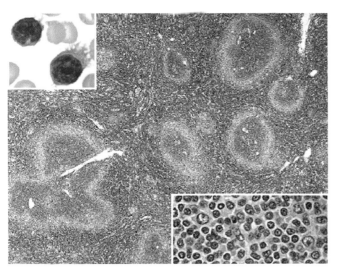

Fig 8.8 Splenic marginal zone lymphoma.

MARGINAL ZONE B CELL LYMPHOMA, EXTRANODAL (MALT TYPE)

Marginal zone lymphomas (Fig. 8.6) are thought to represent the neoplastic equivalent of the marginal zone cells found in the spleen and lymph nodes. The only marginal zone neoplasm unequivocally recognized in the REAL scheme is a small cell lymphoma. This arises in the gastrointestinal tract or other extranodal sites, usually glandular epithelial tissues, and is commonly referred to as 'MALT lymphoma'. These neoplasms derive from the B cells associated with epithelial tissues, and usually arise against a background of reactive lymphoid tissue, in which non-neoplastic germinal centres are prominent. They tend to remain localized, so that their prognosis is usually good, but they can transform to a large cell B cell lymphoma. When they spread to local lymph nodes the appearance is identical to that of the rare 'monocytoid' B cell lymphoma.

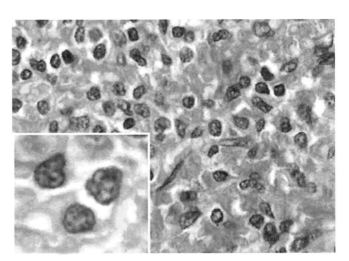

Fig 8.7 Hairy cell leukaemia.

SPLENIC MARGINAL ZONE LYMPHOMA

Splenic marginal zone lymphoma (Fig. 8.8) was included in the REAL scheme as a provisional entity, even though it is not certain that the neoplasm arises from marginal zone cells in the spleen. A major difference from marginal zone lymphoma of MALT type is the high incidence of bone marrow disease at presentation. It almost certainly corresponds to the disease recognized by haematologists as 'splenic lymphoma with villous lymphocytes', a rare form of chronic leukaemia.

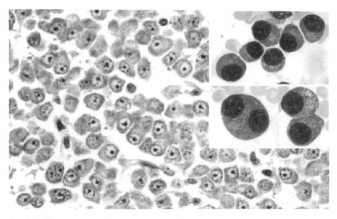

Fig 8.9 Plasmacytoma/plasma cell myeloma.

PLASMACYTOMA/PLASMA CELL MYELOMA
Plasma cells are the cells characteristic of myeloma or plasmacytoma (Fig. 8.9), the former term being used when the neoplasm is found in the bone marrow, causing skeletal destruction, and the latter for the rarer tumours that arise in soft tissue. B cell surface antigens are generally absent, in keeping with their loss by normal mature plasma cells, but cytoplasmic Ig (of a single light chain type) is present, accompanied in about 50% of cases by CD79a, one of the two chains of the molecule associated with Ig in B cells. The chromosome abnormality characteristic of mantle cell lymphoma (the (11;14) translocation) is found in some cases. Patients with multiple myeloma usually respond initially to therapy, but almost all relapse after a period of remission.

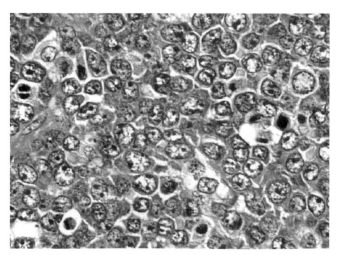

Fig 8.10 Diffuse large B cell lymphoma.

DIFFUSE LARGE B CELL LYMPHOMA
'Diffuse large B cell lymphoma' (Fig. 8.10) was established in the REAL scheme to combine the 'centroblastic' and immunoblastic' categories. It is one of the commonest categories of non-Hodgkin's

lymphoma. Pan-B cell markers are expressed, and in a minority of cases the (14;18) chromosomal translocation is present, suggesting an origin from follicular lymphoma. The disease usually requires aggressive treatment, but may respond well, at least for a period.

The REAL scheme recognizes primary mediastinal (thymic) lymphoma as a rare subtype of large B cell lymphoma. The neoplastic cells often have characteristic pale cytoplasm and are thought to arise from intrathymic B cells and sclerosis is commonly seen and it has distinctive clinical features, e.g. it tends to occur in younger female patients and to relapse at extranodal sites.

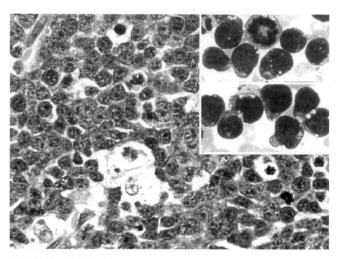

Fig 8.11 Burkitt's lymphoma.

BURKITT'S LYMPHOMA
Burkitt's lymphoma (Fig. 8.11) was originally described in African patients. The tumour is typically made up of medium-sized B cells with a high proliferation fraction, interspersed with macrophages containing cellular debris, giving the characteristic 'starry sky' appearance. It may be difficult to distinguish with certainty from diffuse large cell lymphoma. The immunophenotype is that of a peripheral B cell, although CD10 is also often present, which has prompted suggestions that it derives from germinal centre cells. In most of these 'endemic' African cases Epstein Barr viral DNA is found in the malignant cells. Histologically and phenotypically identical cases are also seen in the West. These may arise in patients with AIDS, and the EB virus is also detectable in almost half of these cases. Non-African 'sporadic' cases also arise in the absence of immune impairment and EB virus is detectable in less than a quarter of these cases. Almost all cases, from whatever country, show a chromosomal translocation involving the *MYC* gene on chromosome 8 and the gene for Ig heavy chain or, less commonly, one of the two Ig light chain genes. The disease may respond to aggressive therapy.

Precursor T cell neoplasms
Precursor T lymphoblastic leukaemia/lymphoma

Peripheral T cell and NK cell neoplasms
T cell chronic lymphocytic leukaemia/prolymphocytic leukaemia
Large granular lymphocyte leukaemia (LGL)
Mycosis fungoides/Sézary syndrome
Peripheral T cell lymphomas, unspecified
Angioimmunoblastic T cell lymphoma (AILD)
Angiocentric lymphoma (nasal NK/T cell lymphoma)
Intestinal T cell lymphoma
Adult T cell lymphoma/leukaemia (ATL/L)
Anaplastic large cell lymphoma (ALCL)

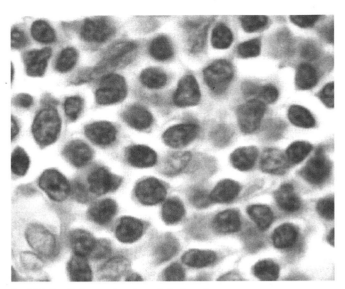

Fig 8.13 T cell chronic lymphocytic leukaemia.

T CELL AND NATURAL KILLER CELL NEOPLASMS IN THE REAL CLASSIFICATION

The other major category of lymphoid neoplasia in the REAL scheme (apart from Hodgkin's disease) comprises those arising from T cell or natural killer cells. As in the case of the B cell disorders, they are subdivided into lymphoblastic neoplasms, which arise from immature cells of thymic origin, and those which arise from mature peripheral T cells.

T CELL CHRONIC LYMPHOCYTIC LEUKAEMIA (FIG. 8.13)

T cell lymphomas of small lymphocytes resemble small lymphocytic B cell neoplasms in that they often involve the peripheral blood, and their morphology is similar. Generally their nucleoli are more prominent and the cytoplasm more abundant, so that the cells would be classified haematologically as 'prolymphocytes'. Unlike small lymphocytic B cell lymphoma, pseudofollicles containing larger cells are not seen. This category includes what haematologists categorize as T cell prolymphocytic leukaemia. These lymphomas express pan-T cell antigens and also CD7, and are commonly CD4-positive. The disease tends to follow a rather more aggressive course than small lymphocytic B cell tumours.

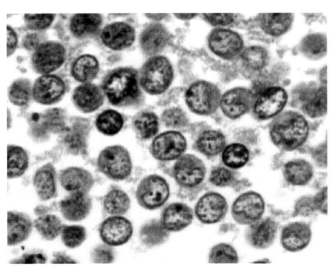

Fig 8.12 T lymphoblastic leukaemia/lymphoma.

T LYMPHOBLASTIC LEUKAEMIA/LYMPHOMA

The morphology of lymphoblastic neoplasms of precursor T cell origin is usually indistinguishable from that of B cell lymphoblastic neoplasms (Fig. 8.12). They typically present as acute leukaemias but occasionally give rise to tumours in the lymph node or thymus. T cell antigens are present although CD3 is usually, because of the immaturity of the cells, only found in the cytoplasm. The disease is potentially curable with aggressive therapy.

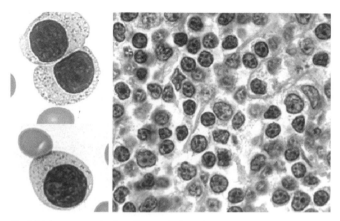

Fig 8.14 Large granular lymphocyte leukaemia.

PERIPHERAL T CELL LYMPHOMA, UNSPECIFIED

The REAL scheme created a single category of 'peripheral T cell lymphoma' (Fig. 8.15) because of the lack of reproducibility amongst pathologists of the subtypes recognized by the Kiel classification. The word 'unspecified' was added to indicate that it may comprise a number of different entities.

These neoplasms typically contain a mixture of small and large neoplastic cells, often with irregular nuclei. There may be a marked infiltration of non-neoplastic cells, including macrophages and eosinophils. In some cases, clusters of epithelioid histiocytes, characteristic of so-called 'Lennert's' or lymphoepithelioid T cell lymphoma, are seen. A variety of patterns of T cell antigen expression is found, CD4 being more frequent than CD8. Peripheral T cell lymphomas are for some reason seen with greater frequency in the Far East than in Europe and the United States, where they account for less than 20% of non-Hodgkin's lymphomas. The prognosis is very variable.

LARGE GRANULAR LYMPHOCYTE LEUKAEMIA

Neoplasms arising from 'large granular lymphocytes' present most frequently as a haematological disorder, in which 'Tγ lymphocytosis' is associated with neutropenia (Fig. 8.14). A proportion of patients have clinical features of rheumatoid arthritis, and an unclear relationship exists with cases of Felty's syndrome. They can be subdivided, on the basis of phenotype, into those which arise from T cells and those which derive from natural killer cells.

The disease is usually indolent, although the course tends to be more aggressive in Asian cases, in which the neoplastic cells are of natural killer type and contain Epstein Barr viral DNA. The borderline is not always clear between these Asian cases and angiocentric lymphomas.

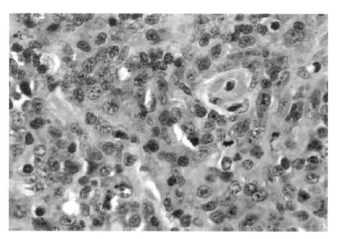

Fig 8.15 Peripheral T cell lymphoma, unspecified.

MYCOSIS FUNGOIDES/SÉZARY SYNDROME

Mycosis fungoides is a T cell lymphoma arising in the skin, but which is referred to as Sézary syndrome when the lymphoma cells are also found in the circulation (Fig. 8.16). The neoplastic cells accumulate in the epidermis, where they may form localized pockets referred to as 'Pautrier's micro-abscesses', and have a typical highly convoluted cerebriform nuclear morphology. As the disease progresses it can spread to lymph nodes, where the interfollicular zones are infiltrated. The cells express pan-T cell antigens and are almost always of CD4 or 'helper' subtype. In many cases a number of the neoplastic T cells also express CD30 which can be a useful feature to distinguish it from dermatitis. The disease follows a variable course but may become widespread and has a tendency to transform to a large cell tumour.

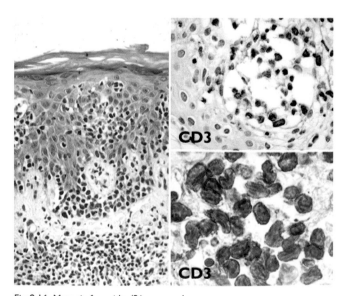

Fig 8.16 Mycosis fungoides/Sézary syndrome.

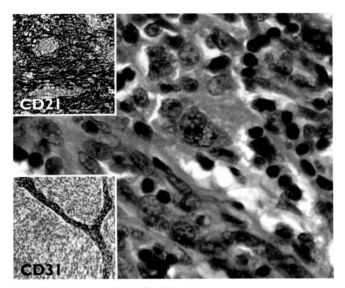

Fig 8.17 Angioimmunoblastic T cell lymphoma.

INTESTINAL T CELL LYMPHOMA (FIG. 8.18)

Small intestinal lymphomas have long been recognized as a complication of coeliac disease. They were first thought to be a heterogeneous group of tumours but later studies suggested a histiocytic origin. In the early 1980s it became clear that they were T cell lymphomas of widely varying morphology. This neoplasm is often associated with small bowel ulceration. The typical histological features of coeliac disease, though often present, may be absent due to the phenomenon of 'latency' recently recognized in coeliac patients. In keeping with this, some patients have a history of documented coeliac disease while others present with the lymphoma. The neoplastic cells express pan T cell markers and, in most cases, the CD103 integrin molecule found on normal intestinal T lymphocytes. The clinical outlook is poor since the neoplasm is often multifocal.

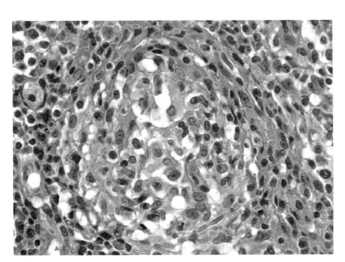

Fig 8.19 Angiocentric lymphoma.

ANGIOIMMUNOBLASTIC T CELL LYMPHOMA

Angioimmunoblastic T cell lymphoma (Fig. 8.17) was initially thought of as an abnormal immune reaction, but is now considered as a category of peripheral T cell lymphoma in which the neoplastic cells are mixed with and obscured by a complex histological picture including proliferating vessels, epithelioid histiocytes, plasma cells, eosinophils, and hyperplastic clusters of follicular dendritic cells. The neoplastic cells are of variable morphology and include atypical 'clear' cells with round nuclei and abundant pale cytoplasm. The cells carry T cell markers and are usually CD4-positive. Patients often have systemic symptoms such as weight loss, fever, skin rash and a polyclonal hypergammaglobulinemia. The disease is moderately aggressive and a high grade lymphoma (usually of T but occasionally of B cell type) may emerge.

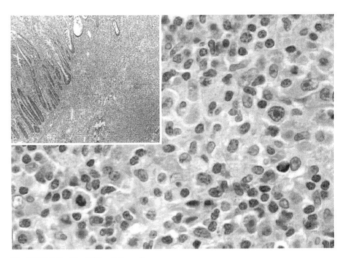

Fig 8.18 Intestinal T cell lymphoma.

ANGIOCENTRIC LYMPHOMA

This is an extranodal lymphoma involving the nose, upper airways and soft tissues (Fig. 8.19). There is a tendency to invade the walls of blood vessels, accompanied in many cases by blockage of vessels by lymphoma cells, often associated with ischaemic necrosis of normal and neoplastic tissue. The origin of the neoplastic cells is unclear: T cell antigens can be present, but CD3 is absent in many cases and CD56, a molecule associated with natural killer cells, is often expressed. The disease is rare in the United States and Europe, but is much commoner in Asia. The distinction from Asian neoplasms of large granular lymphocytes is not always clear. The disease may be curable if localized but disseminated cases have a poor prognosis.

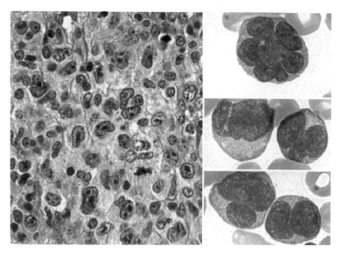

Fig 8.20 Adult T cell lymphoma/leukaemia.

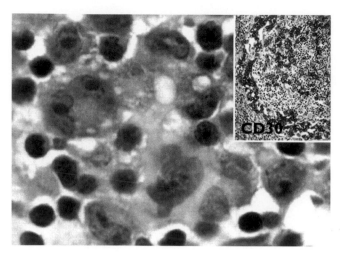

Fig 8.21 Anaplastic large cell lymphoma.

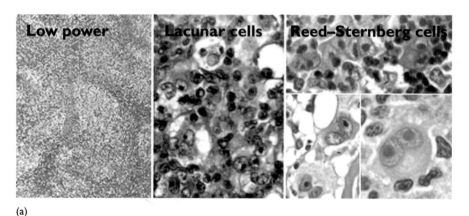

(a)

Fig 8.22 (a) Hodgkin's disease, nodular sclerosis.

ADULT T CELL LYMPHOMA/LEUKAEMIA (FIG. 8.20)

In the 1970s, an unusual T cell neoplasm was reported in South Western Japan which was subsequently shown to be confined to patients infected with the HTLV-1 retrovirus. Identical cases were then found in other areas of HTLV-1 infection, notably the Caribbean. The lymph node is diffusely replaced by neoplastic T cells, which vary widely in cell size and shape, and neoplastic cells may also be seen in the peripheral blood. Patients often have aggressive disease, associated with lytic bone lesions, and hypercalcaemia, but the course is very variable, and indolent or smouldering cases are seen.

ANAPLASTIC LARGE CELL LYMPHOMA

Anaplastic large cell lymphoma (Fig. 8.21) was first recognized as a neoplasm which was positive for the Ki-1 or CD30 antigen, an activation-associated antigen also found on Reed–Sternberg cells. The neoplastic cells can be larger than in any other type of lymphoma, and cases may be misdiagnosed as malignant histiocytosis or even anaplastic carcinoma. Distinction from Hodgkin's disease may also on occasion be difficult. Typically the tumour grows in a cohesive pattern, tending to invade lymphoid sinuses, and may spread to soft tissue, bone and skin. The neoplasm may be negative for cell lineage markers, but if such antigens are present, they commonly indicate a T cell origin. In some cases there is a translocation between chromosome 2 and 5, causing fusion of the nucleophosmin gene with a novel gene encoding the ALK receptor kinase. Patients can be of all ages and at least 50% of cases are seen in children or young adults. The clinical pattern is variable, some cases showing widespread involvement of lymph nodes and other sites and other cases tending to be confined to skin. The latter form of the disease is indolent but difficult to cure, whereas the systemic type may respond to aggressive treatment.

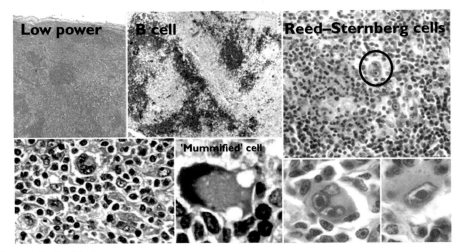

Fig 8.22(b) Hodgkin's disease, mixed cellularity.

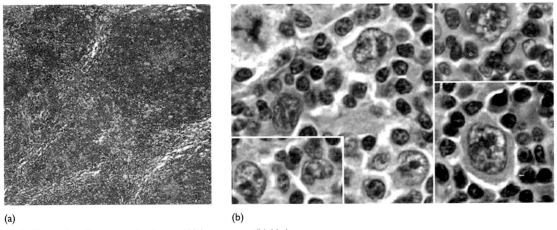

(a)   (b)

Fig 8.23 Hodgkin's disease, lymphocyte predominance. (a) Low power. (b) High power.

Hodgkin's disease – classical subtypes

In classical Hodgkin's disease, scattered binucleate or multinucleate Reed–Sternberg cells and mononuclear Hodgkin's cells are seen, associated with a reactive cellular infiltrate of lymphoid cells, eosinophils and other inflammatory cells (Fig. 8.22(a)). The nodular sclerosis subtype is characterized by prominent fibrotic bands running through the diseased tissue, a thickened lymph node capsule and 'lacunar' cells, a peculiar variant of the Reed–Sternberg cell. These features are absent in mixed cellularity Hodgkin's disease, in which the heterogeneous cellular infiltrate is the cardinal feature. When this infiltrate is sparse and Reed–Sternberg cells numerous and often bizarre, the disease falls into the lymphocyte depletion category, while the reverse pattern is seen in the provisional lymphocyte rich category. The lymphocyte depletion subtype is rare and may be difficult to distinguish from anaplastic large cell lymphoma.

Hodgkin's disease – mixed cellularity

In mixed cellularity Hodgkin's disease the node is uniformly replaced by a mixed infiltrate of abnormal and reactive cells (Fig. 8.22(b)). The infiltrate usually has a paracortical localization, as seen when remnants of follicles are demonstrated by immunostaining for B cell antigens. When this pattern is marked, a diagnosis is sometimes made of 'interfollicular' Hodgkin's disease. Apoptotic or 'mummified' neoplastic cells are commonly found.

Lymphocyte predominance

Lymphocyte predominance Hodgkin's disease (Fig. 8.23) shares with the classical subtypes of Hodgkin's disease a histological picture in which scattered neoplastic cells are seen against the background of an abnormal cellular infiltrate. However most of the neoplastic cells, known as 'L & H' (lymphocytic and histiocytic) or 'popcorn' cells, lie within large nodular areas made up of small lymphoid cells.

Reference

1 Lee Harris N, Jaffe ES, Stein H, Banks PM, Chan JKC, Cleary ML, Delsol G, De Wolf-Peeters C, Falini B, Gatter KC, Grogan TM, Isaacson PG, Knowles DM, Mason DY, Müller-Hermelink H-K, Pileri SA, Piris MA, Ralfkiaer E and Warnke RA. A Revised European American classification of lymphoid neoplasms: A proposal from the international lymphoma study group. *Blood* 1994; **84**; 1361–1392.

Acute lymphoblastic leukaemia and lymphoma

Chapter 8.2

General features

These neoplasms may be of B (mainly the so-called pre-B) or T cell type. Much discussion and argument has gone on about the relationship between acute lymphoblastic leukaemia (ALL) and lymphoblastic lymphoma though most of it is of little assistance when examining trephines. Most cases that present with bone marrow involvement, whether or not there is tissue infiltration, are of B cell type. The T cell lymphoblastics are rarer (less than 20% of all lymphoblastic lymphomas in most series) but give rise to the well-described clinical syndrome of mediastinal tumours without an obvious leukaemic phase. Lymphoblastic lesions are aggressive and are rapidly fatal if untreated. With current treatment they are potentially curable, especially in the younger age group with ALL.

Histopathology of the bone marrow

B and T cell cases have identical morphological features. The neoplastic lymphoblasts are slightly larger than lymphocytes and have round or convoluted nuclei, fine chromatin often with a smudged appearance, inconspicuous nucleoli and scant, faintly basophilic cytoplasm. Mitotic figures are numerous (Fig. 8.24). The marrow is packed with little of the haematopoietic tissue or fat remaining though occasionally a more patchy infiltration is evident (Fig. 8.25). Areas of necrosis (often a sinister sign in a marrow) may be present. The distinction between B and T cell cases can only be made immunocytochemically (Fig. 8.26). An important practical note is that B lymphoblasts have a precursor phenotype being CD79a positive but usually lacking mature B markers such as CD20.

Immunophenotype B cell: TdT+, CD10+/-, CD19+, CD20-, CD22-, CD79a+, SIg-
Immunophenotype T cell: TdT+, CD3+, CD7+, CD2 & 5 variable, CD4+/-, CD8+/-

---

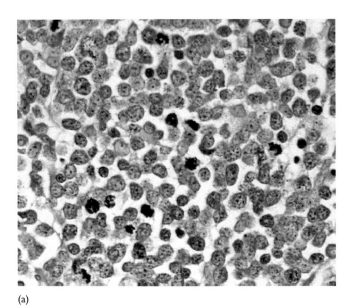
(a)

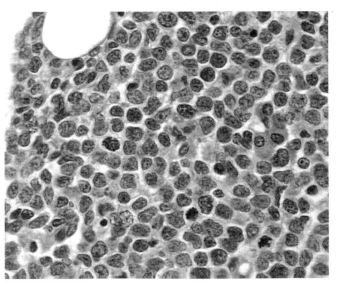
(b)

Fig 8.24 Cytology of lymphoblastic lymphoma. (a) Giemsa. (b) H&E.

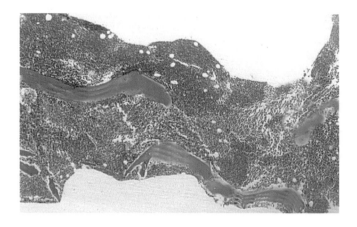

Fig 8.25 Hypercellular marrow in lymphoblastic lymphoma. H&E.

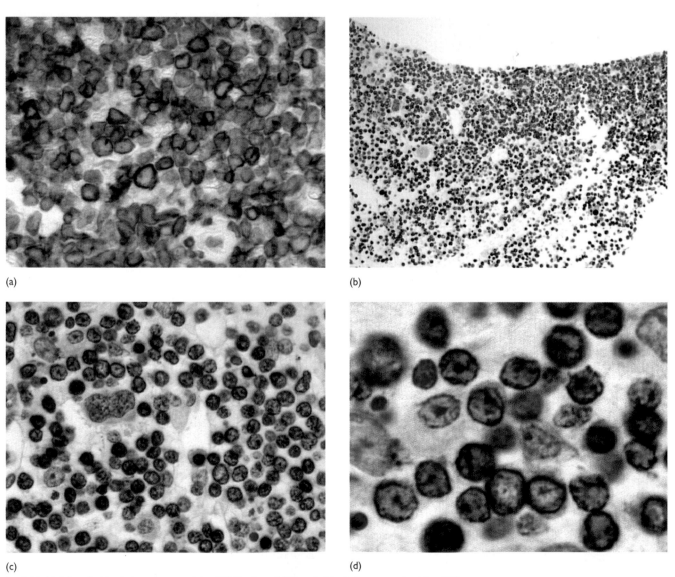

(a)

(b)

(c)

(d)

Fig 8.26 (a) B lymphoblastic immunostained for CD79a. (b – d) T lymphoblastic immunostained for CD3.

Diagnostic problems

1 Sparse infiltrate

Occasionally the infiltrate is sparse with blast cells outnumbered by normal marrow cells so that it is easy for the histologist to overlook them. This may occur at diagnosis as well as at early relapse and is relatively easily recognized by immunostaining for B or T cell antigens (Fig. 8.27).

2 Distinction from CLL

The small size of the lymphoblasts and the packed nature of the marrow can produce a picture in an adult which is surprisingly easy to confuse with CLL, although this does not seem to have been admitted in print. It can be avoided by checking for a high mitotic rate in ALL which will be confirmed by abundant positively stained nuclei for proliferation markers such as Ki67 (Fig. 8.28).

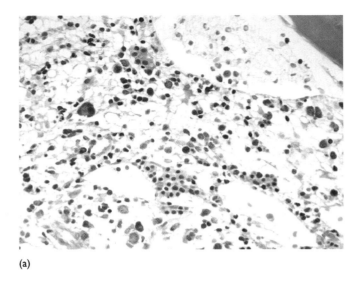

(a)

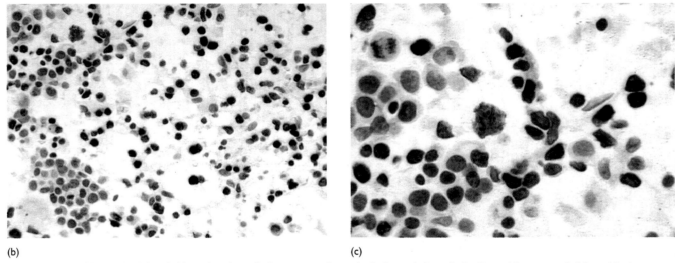

(b)

(c)

Fig 8.27 Scanty infiltration by B lymphoblastic lymphoma/leukaemia is easily overlooked morphologically (a: Giemsa) but is revealed (b – c) by immunostaining for CD79a.

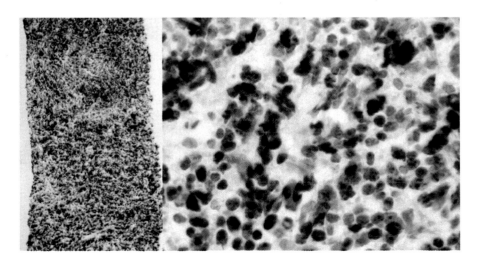

Fig 8.28 Immunostain for Ki67, low power (left) and high power (right), showing high proliferative activity in lymphoblastic lymphoma.

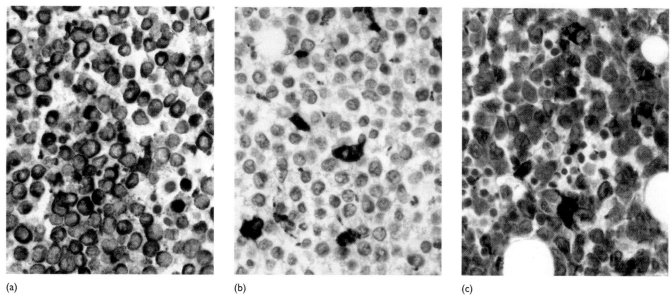

(a) (b) (c)

Fig 8.29 Typical immunostains for AML show (a) M1 myeloperoxidase positive but (b) CD68 negative whereas (c) an M5 case is strongly CD68 positive.

3 Distinction from AML

Histologically AML (M0-5) looks like ALL. The only currently available distinction is the recognition of ALL by B and T cell or AML by myeloid associated immunostaining (Fig. 8.29).

Summary of key points
- Aggressive but potentially curable disease.
- Small blast cells with high mitotic rate.
- Packed marrow (often virtually a total replacement).
- May resemble CLL at low power.

Chronic lymphocytic leukaemia (CLL)/small lymphocytic lymphoma

Chapter 8.3

General features

The separation of small lymphocytic lymphoma and chronic lymphocytic leukaemia (CLL) is arbitrary and is based on the tissue involved, i.e. blood, bone marrow or lymphoid organs. Some patients may have disease restricted to one site though the majority will show evidence of marrow involvement. It should be remembered that the neoplastic cell is morphologically and immunophenotypically identical in all of these settings. It is for this reason that major lymphoma classifications such as REAL or Kiel use the term CLL for all aspects of this disease.

The neoplastic cell is usually (99%) a B cell. The rare T cell variant is difficult to recognize on cell morphology alone.

Clinical

This is the most frequent leukaemia in Europe and North America. It is more common in men and the median age at diagnosis is 60 years. Patients may present with tiredness, breathlessness, enlarged lymph nodes and in the later stages with bleeding problems and infections. Mild to moderate hepatosplenomegaly may be present.

In T cell CLL skin involvement may occur. In prolymphocytic leukaemia splenomegaly is often marked but lymphadenopathy is uncommon.

Histopathology of the bone marrow

Marrow involved by CLL is generally hypercellular. Residual marrow elements are usually present unless the disease is advanced in which case the marrow spaces are packed with the neoplastic cells. Several patterns of involvement have been described, i.e. interstitial, nodular, mixed (interstitial and nodular) and diffuse. These patterns recognize marrow involvement at different stages of disease progression.

The most frequent pattern at presentation is mixed. The marrow contains aggregates of the neoplastic cells and also has a background infiltrate throughout the marrow intimately admixed with the haematopoietic tissue. The aggregates usually have a central distribution within the marrow space (Fig. 8.30) although as they increase in size they will eventually expand into contact with the endosteum (Fig. 8.31).

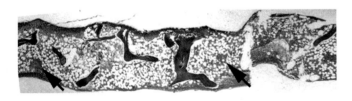

(a)

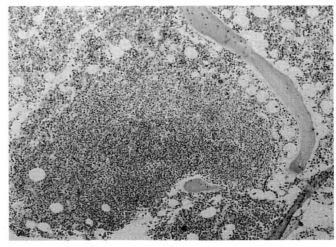

(b)

Fig 8.30 Early presentation of CLL with small centrally located nodules (arrows). (a) Low power. (b) Medium power.

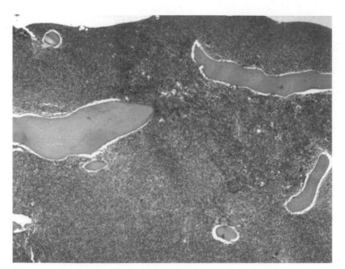

Fig 8.31 Hypercellular packed marrow of advanced CLL. H&E.

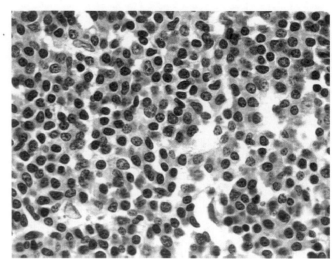

Fig 8.32 (a)

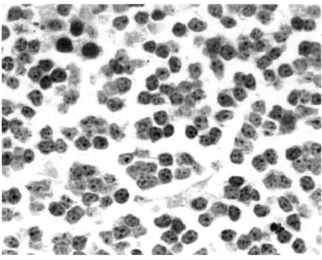

(b)

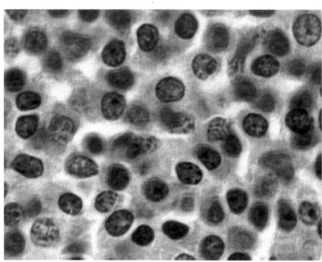

(c)

Fig 8.32 Cytological appearances of CLL in bone marrow sections. (a – c) Giemsa.

The neoplastic cell is a small lymphocyte with a round nucleus, clumped chromatin and inconspicuous nucleolus (Fig. 8.32).

The proliferation centres, containing larger prolymphocytes and paraimmunoblasts that are an obvious part of nodal disease are occasionally seen in the bone marrow (Fig. 8.33).

One distinguishing feature of T cell CLL is that it does not form proliferation centres.

In patients with peripheral destruction of platelets in enlarged spleens it is possible to see a reactive hyperplasia of the megakaryocytic series in the bone marrow.

Richter's syndrome, the transformation of CLL to a large cell lymphoma, occurs in a small proportion of cases (Fig. 8.34).

Immunophenotype: CD19+, CD20+, CD79a+, CD5+, CD23+, CD43+

Variations such as prolymphocytic leukaemia are more reliably identified on smears. These patients have more aggressive disease and respond less well to the treatment regimes used for CLL. Prolymphocytes, which must form more than half the neoplastic cell population, have a prominent central nucleolus and more cytoplasm than CLL cells (Fig. 8.35).

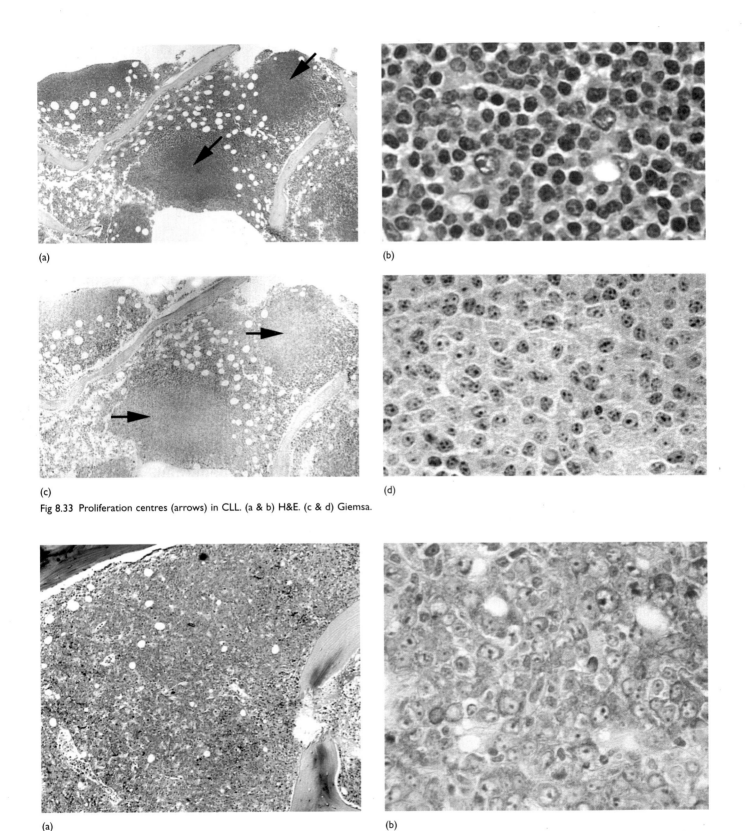

(a)

(b)

(c)

(d)

Fig 8.33 Proliferation centres (arrows) in CLL. (a & b) H&E. (c & d) Giemsa.

(a)

(b)

Fig 8.34 Richter's syndrome: a large cell lymphoma has arisen in the marrow of a patient previously showing typical CLL. (a & b) Low and high power.

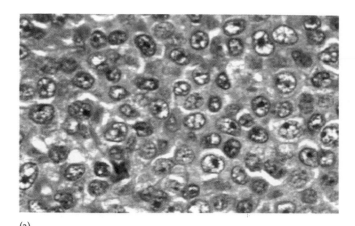

(a)

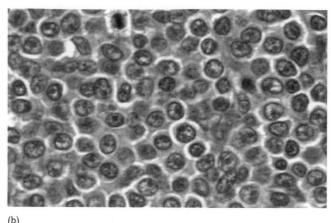

(b)

Fig 8.35 The appearances of prolymphocytic leukaemia cells in bone marrow trephine sections from two separate cases.

Many cases of CLL show a degree of plasmacytic differentiation yet have the same immunophenotype as typical CLL. There does not appear to be any difference in the clinical behaviour of these cases from typical CLL. These cases were separately classified in the Kiel scheme as lymphoplasmacytoid lymphoma but have been considered to be the same entity in the REAL classification. They differ from immunocytoma (Waldenström's macroglobulinaemia) both morphologically and immunophenotypically.

Diagnostic problems
Distinction between reactive lymphoid nodules and CLL
In CLL the number of nodules is usually more than three in a trephine of >1 cm in length, although confirmation of clonality may be needed to confirm the diagnosis. Other histological features which may be helpful have been discussed previously (see Chapter 2).

Is it possible to distinguish between CLL and small cell lymphocytic lymphoma on marrow histology?
There are no definite features which allow a reliable distinction to be made.

Distinguishing between cytopenias which are immune based and those due to loss of haematopoietic tissue
Some patients with CLL develop cytopenias. In those cases where this is due to loss of haematopoietic tissue the marrow will show replacement of the normal blood-forming cell lines by malignant cells. In those cases where the cytopenias are immune-based and the blood cells are being destroyed, a hyperplastic picture may be seen with the affected cell lines displaying increased numbers of their more immature members in an attempt to replace the cells destroyed peripherally.

Distinguishing between CLL and small cell acute leukaemias
On histology alone it is surprisingly easy to misdiagnose ALL as CLL especially in an adult where the former is unexpected. Full knowledge of the clinical picture and close inspection of the cell morphology will prevent such a mistake (although it is unlikely one would get such a howler past a competent haematologist!). Mitotic figures will be obvious in acute leukaemia and virtually absent in CLL.

Summary of key points
- This is a low-grade, indolent lymphoma although it is currently incurable.
- The majority are B cell.
- The marrow is hypercellular and usually has a nodular pattern.
- The nodules have a central, inter-trabecular distribution.
- CLL variants are difficult to identify on marrow histology.

Immunocytoma including Waldenström's macroglobulinaemia

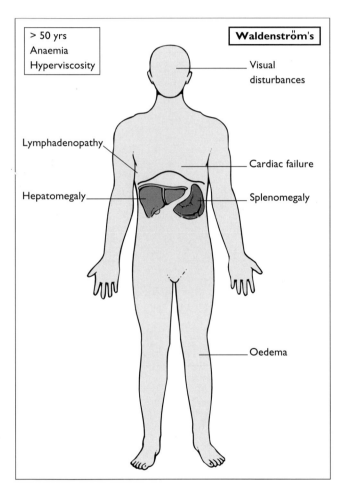

Fig 8.36 Clinical features of immunocytoma.

General features

This low-grade B cell malignancy shows a particular tendency towards plasma cell differentiation. Although commonly lymph-node-based it may present in the bone marrow when it is often associated with the clinical syndrome of Waldenström's macroglob-ulinaemia. This is characterized by an IgM paraprotein in the serum. These patients usually present with increasing tiredness. The large IgM protein molecules increase the blood's viscosity, producing visual disturbances and cardiac failure. There is often lymphadenopathy and hepatosplenomegaly (Fig. 8.36).

Histopathology of the bone marrow

At presentation the marrow is often hypocellular (Fig. 8.37) but becomes increasingly infiltrated as the disease progresses. The normal haematopoietic tissue is replaced by neoplastic B cells

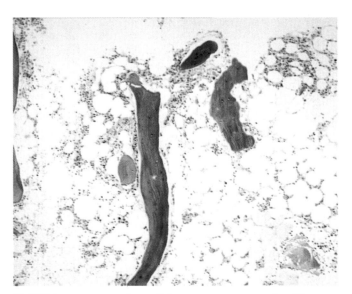

Fig 8.37 Immunocytoma: hypocellular marrow at presentation. Giemsa.

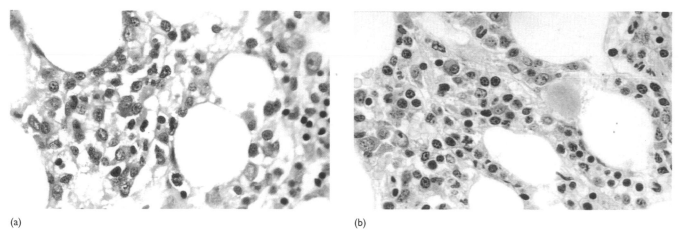

(a)   (b)

Fig 8.38 Immunocytoma is composed of a range of cells from lymphocytes to plasma cells. (a) H&E. (b) Giemsa.

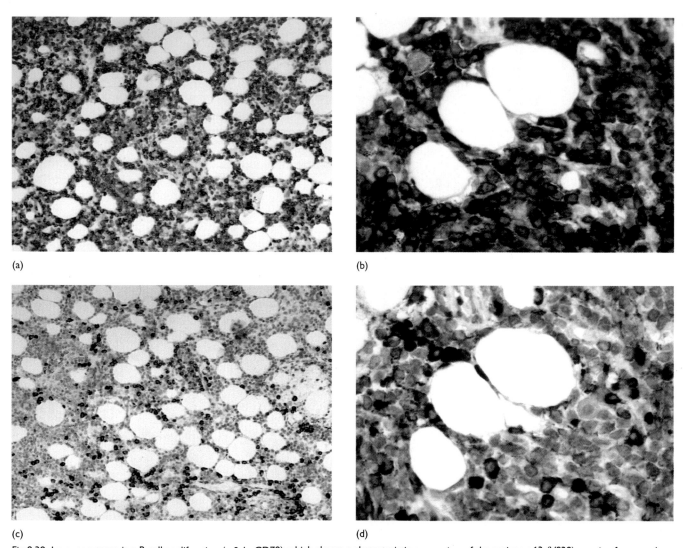

(a)   (b)

(c)   (d)

Fig 8.39 Immunocytoma is a B cell proliferation (a & b: CD79) which shows a characteristic expression of the antigen p63 (VS38), ranging from weak on lymphoid to strong on plasma cells. (c & d) Immunostain for p63 (VS38).

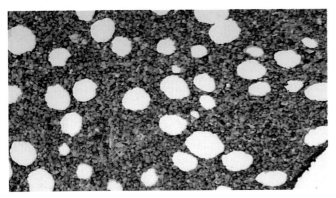

Fig 8.40 Kappa light chain restriction in an immunocytoma.

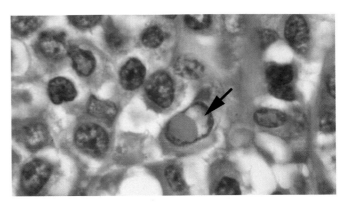

Fig 8.41 Dutcher body (arrow) in an immunocytoma.

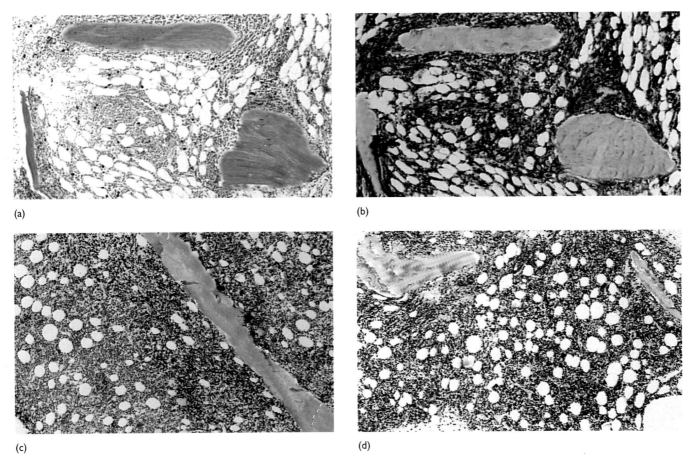

(a)

(b)

(c)

(d)

Fig 8.42 Infiltration of the bone marrow by immunocytoma showing both paratrabecular and central involvement. (a) Giemsa. (b) CD79a (B cell). (c & d) VS38 (p63).

showing a range of differentiation between lymphocytes and plasma cells (Fig. 8.38) which appropriate immunostains will highlight dramatically. In fact the differential expression of a plasma cell marker such as VS38 (p63) can be very effective in differentiating immunocytoma from other B cell lymphomas (with little positivity) and myeloma (where all neoplastic cells are positive) (Fig. 8.39).

IgM and light chain restriction can be demonstrated immunohistochemically in the neoplastic cells (Fig. 8.40).

Some of the plasmacytoid cells and plasma cells contain perinuclear accumulations of IgM which indent the nucleus and appear to be intranuclear (Dutcher bodies) (Fig. 8.41).

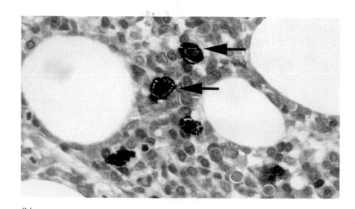

(a)
(b)

Fig 8.43 Mast cells (arrows) in a case of immunocytoma giving rise to Waldenström's macroglobulinaemia. Giemsa.

Early involvement is frequently patchy, sometimes resembling CLL with centrally located nodules and at other times follicular lymphoma with paratrabecular aggregations. There is also a sparse diffuse infiltrate spreading through the rest of the marrow easily seen with immunocytochemical assistance (Fig. 8.42). As the disease progresses this enlarges to fill the entire marrow.

Two additional features may be seen in association with the neoplastic cell infiltrate.

1 Mast cells are often numerous. They are best seen in a Giemsa-stained section as this reveals the metachromatic properties of the cell's granules. Although these cells are increased in a number of other lymphoproliferative conditions which affect the bone marrow, they are particularly numerous in Waldenström's macroglobulinaemia (Fig. 8.43).

2 Within the interstitium there is deposition of an amorphous, eosinophilic, PAS-positive substance, probably IgM (Fig. 8.44).

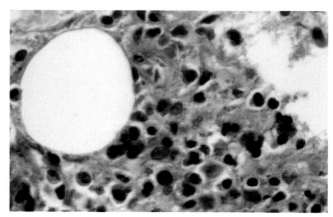

Fig 8.44 Interstitial deposition of presumed IgM in a case of Waldenström's macroglobulinaemia. PAS.

Immunophenotype: positive for surface and cytoplasmic Ig (usually IgM), CD19, CD20, CD22, CD79a. They lack CD5, CD10. The strong cytoplasmic Ig staining and lack of CD5 help distinguish it from B-CLL.

Summary of key points
- The neoplastic cells have features of both small lymphocytes and plasma cells.
- The neoplastic cells produce cytoplasmic Ig (usually IgM) and lack CD5.
- Mast cells are often very prominent.

Mantle cell lymphoma (MCL)

Chapter 8.5

General features

This is known as centrocytic lymphoma by the Kiel group who originally described it. Prior to this it had been regarded by many as a lymphoma showing differentiation intermediate between CLL and follicular lymphoma. The neoplastic cells are now believed to originate from the mantle zone and not from the germinal centre. Many cases have a t(11;14) translocation which appears to activate cyclin D1 (this is a cell cycle protein not usually expressed in lymphoid cells). Cyclin D1 is also raised in cases without this translocation, indicating that other mechanisms may also be involved.

It generally occurs in adults over 50 years, often male, and is usually widespread at diagnosis. It involves lymph nodes, spleen, Waldeyer's ring, bone marrow and the gastro-intestinal tract (lymphomatous polyposis). It has a more aggressive course than other low grade lymphomas and is currently incurable (Fig. 8.45).

It does not seem to transform to large cell lymphoma but a small to medium-sized blast cell variant may occur which has an even worse prognosis.

Histopathology of the bone marrow

The marrow infiltrate consists of a uniform population of small to medium lymphoid cells with cleaved or angular nuclei, dispersed chromatin, inconspicuous nucleoli and scanty cytoplasm (Fig. 8.46).

Unlike follicular lymphoma virtually no larger cells, i.e. centroblasts, are present. Marrow involvement may be both paratrabecular and diffuse (Fig. 8.47).

> **Immunophenotype:** positive for surface IgM, CD19, 20, 22, 79a, CD5, CD43 and cyclin D1 and negative for CD23.

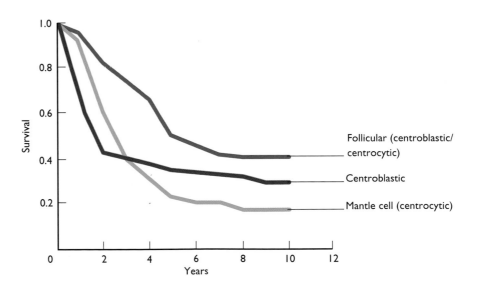

Fig 8.45 Mantle cell lymphoma survival curve.

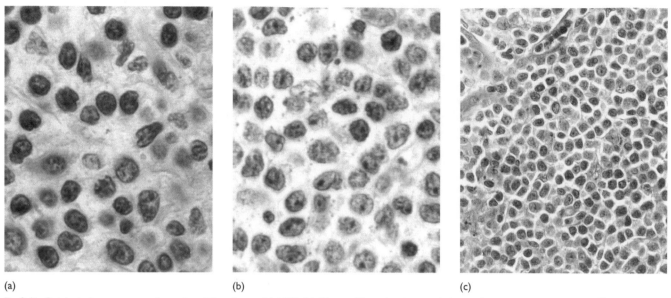

(a)   (b)   (c)

Fig 8.46 Cytological appearances of mantle cell lymphoma. (a) H&E. (b) Giemsa. Note the characteristic grey low-power appearance on Giemsa staining (c).

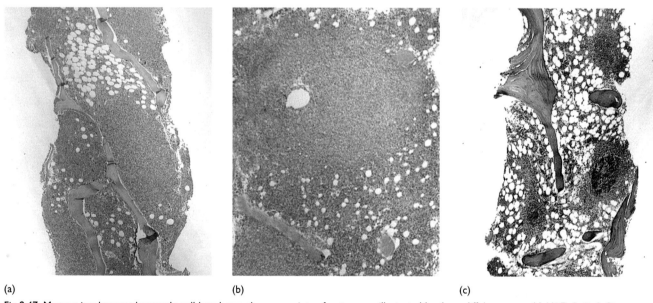

(a)   (b)   (c)

Fig 8.47 Marrow involvement by mantle cell lymphoma shows a variety of patterns as illustrated by three different cases. (a) H&E. (b & c) Giemsa.

Table 8.2 Differential diagnosis of small B cell lymphoma.

	CLL	Follicular lymphoma	MCL
CD5	+	-	+
CD23	+	-/+	-
Cyclin D1	-	-	+

A small number of cases (blastoid variant) have cells with slightly larger nuclei, more dispersed chromatin and a higher proliferation index and to some extent resemble lymphoblasts (Fig. 8.48).

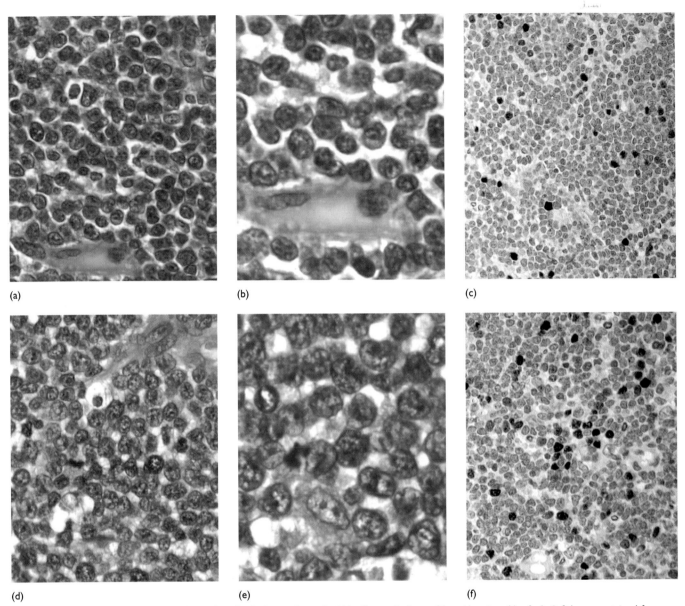

(a)   (b)   (c)

(d)   (e)   (f)

Fig 8.48 Typical case of mantle cell lymphoma (a – c) which transformed within 12 months into a blastoid variant (d – f). (c & f) Immunostained for a proliferation-associated antigen.

Diagnostic problems

Distinguishing CLL, follicular lymphoma and MCL is usually achieved in nodal tissue by an examination of the architecture and cell morphology. This is more difficult on a trephine biopsy. Immunohistochemistry for CD5, CD23 and cyclin D1 is particularly useful in distinguishing these tumours (Table 8.2). Currently available antibodies against these markers are not completely reliable on fixed material even with optimal antigen retrieval.

Summary of key points
- Morphologically the neoplastic cell may resemble a centrocyte or lymphocyte.
- MCL has a more aggressive clinical course than most other lymphomas.
- Rare blastoid variants have an even worse prognosis.
- Immunohistochemistry may be required to differentiate between CLL and follicular lymphoma.

Follicular lymphoma

Chapter 8.6

General features

Follicular lymphoma is also known as centroblastic/centrocytic lymphoma in the Kiel classification. The REAL classification uses the term 'follicle center lymphoma, follicular' which also includes a small number of cases which contain only centroblasts in a follicular pattern. Although the majority of cases have a nodular pattern a small number may be diffuse and have been referred to provisionally as 'follicle center lymphoma, diffuse'. Follicular lymphoma is the commonest type of non-Hodgkin's lymphoma in the West and constitutes about one-third of all NHLs.

It affects adults, usually over 40 years old. It predominantly involves lymph nodes but the spleen, bone marrow and occasionally peripheral blood and extranodal sites may be involved. It has a generally indolent though incurable clinical course. Those cases which display a greater degree of follicle formation and have fewer large cells forming the lymphoma population appear to have a better prognosis than those with a less nodular pattern and more large centroblast-like cells. Some cases may transform into a high-grade, diffuse large cell lymphoma.

Histopathology of the bone marrow

These lymphomas are composed of two cell types: centrocytes (cleaved follicle centre cells) and centroblasts (large non-cleaved follicle centre cells). The centrocytes predominate (Fig. 8.49).

The distribution is characteristic. The lymphoma cells are seen to lie against the trabeculae in little 'drifts' which obliterate the first fat space (Fig. 8.50).

In marrows with extensive involvement these infiltrates increase in size and coalesce to fill the marrow space, gradually losing the characteristic paratrabecular pattern. The nodular pattern of growth seen in lymph nodes is rarely as convincing in the bone marrow even when the infiltrate has virtually filled the whole trephine (Fig. 8.51).

It is recognized that follicular lymphoma may undergo transformation into a large cell NHL. Identification of this depends on increased numbers of centroblasts which should constitute more than 50% of the lymphoma cell population.

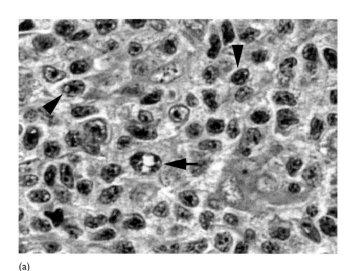

(a)

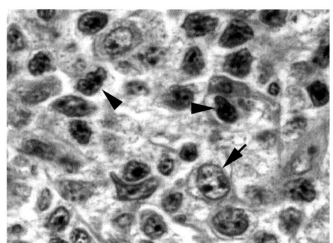

(b)

Fig 8.49 (a & b) Centroblasts (arrow) and centrocytes (arrowheads) in a follicular lymphoma in bone marrow. Giemsa.

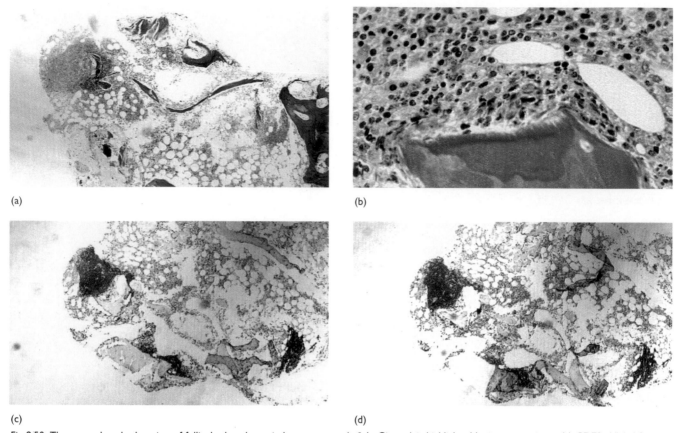

(a)

(b)

(c)

(d)

Fig 8.50 The paratrabecular location of follicular lymphoma in bone marrow (a & b: Giemsa) is highlighted by immunostaining. (c) CD79. (d) bcl-2.

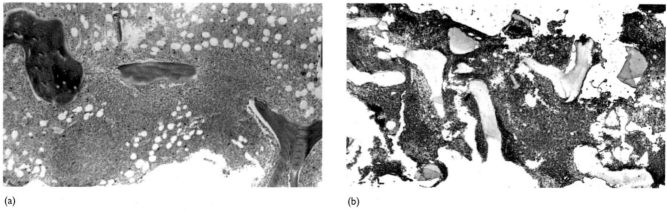

(a)

(b)

Fig 8.51 Extensive infiltration of bone marrow by follicular lymphoma demonstrating both a nodular and diffuse pattern. (a) Giemsa. (b) bcl-2 immuno-stain.

Immunophenotype: surface Ig+, CD19+, CD20+ CD22+, CD79a+, CD10+/-, CD5-, CD23-/+, CD43- and CD11c-

Diagnostic problems

The two main difficulties are in the distinction from reactive nodules and from CLL. In the former the most useful guide is the paratrabecular distribution of follicular lymphoma which does not occur in reactive cases. Although the detection of Bcl-2 protein is

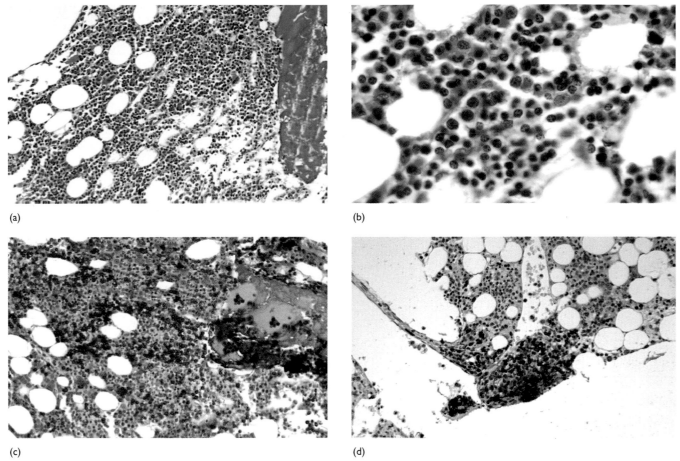

(a)

(b)

(c)

(d)

Fig 8.52 Minimal involvement of the bone marrow by follicular lymphoma may be difficult to detect morphologically (a & b: H&E) but can be readily identified by immunostaining. (c) CD79. (d) bcl-2.

useful in distinguishing reactive from neoplastic nodules in lymph nodes (germinal centres are bcl-2 negative) it is generally not helpful in the marrow since germinal centre formation is rare.

Demonstration of light chain restriction will confirm the diagnosis but this may be difficult on fixed paraffin- or resin-embedded trephines.

Immunocytochemistry is more useful in confirming the diagnosis by showing the typical paratrabecular distribution of the neoplastic B cells which may be virtually invisible to ordinary morphological examination (Fig. 8.52).

This has an additional value in the early stages of marrow involvement by highlighting the affected areas allowing the typical centrocyte morphology of the lymphoma cells to be appreciated (Fig. 8.53).[1]

CLL usually forms round lymphoid aggregates with a central, intertrabecular distribution and is only occasionally paratrabecular.

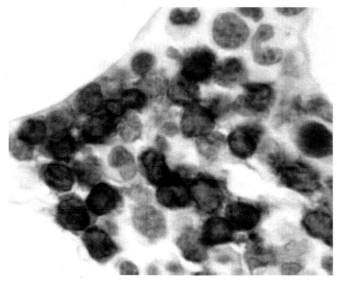

Fig 8.53 Immunostaining allows the abnormal cytology of small deposits of follicular lymphoma to be identified. CD79.

Examination of the nuclear morphology usually allows these two NHLs to be distinguished using conventional stains.

Reference

1 Chetty R, Echezarreta G, Comley M, Gatter K. Immunohistochemistry in apparently normal bone marrow trephine specimens from patients with nodal follicular lymphoma. *J Clin Pathol* 1995; **48**: 1035–1038.

Marginal zone lymphoma (including MALT)

General features

It has become apparent that two recently recognized lymphoma entities, monocytoid B cell lymphoma and the low-grade B cell lymphoma of mucosa-associated lymphoid type (MALT), are probably the same condition with different clinical features. It is believed that the presentation as nodal or extranodal involvement reflects the specific tissue 'homing instincts' of the neoplastic cells. The REAL classification uses the term 'marginal zone lymphoma' to include both extranodal (MALT) and nodal (monocytoid B cell lymphoma) disease.

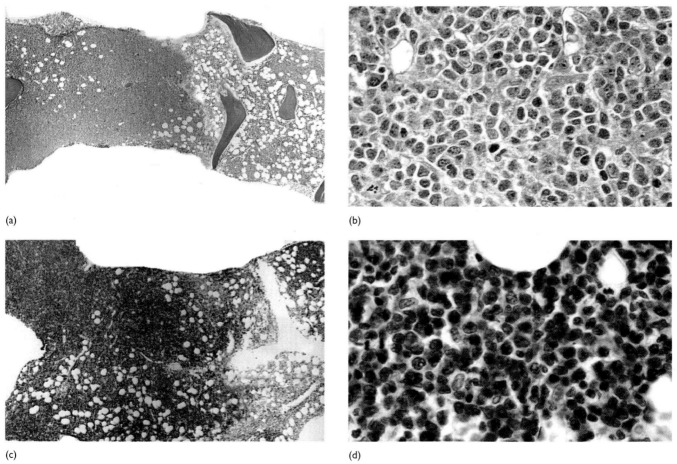

(a)

(b)

(c)

(d)

Fig 8.54 MALT lymphoma in the bone marrow. (a & b) Giemsa. (c & d) CD79 (B cell) immunostain.

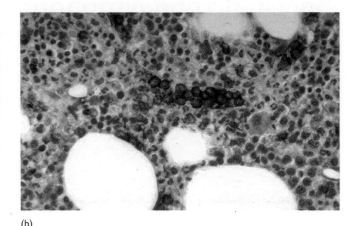

(a)   (b)

Fig. 8.55 Splenic lymphoma involving the bone marrow. (a) H&E. (b) CD20 (B cell immunostain).

Clinically

There are two major clinical presentations.

1 EXTRANODAL. These are tumours of adults and usually involve glandular tissues, most commonly the gastric mucosa where it has been associated with *Helicobacter pylori* gastritis. Disease is often localized and surgical resection may be curative. The clinical course is generally indolent and disseminated disease (e.g. to the bone marrow) is unusual at presentation, and as with other low-grade NHL, is not currently curable. Since the usual association is with glandular tissue the majority of these extranodal marginal zone lymphomas are referred to as MALT lymphomas (or MALTomas). The entity splenic marginal zone lymphoma previously believed to be related to the other marginal zone lymphomas is now known to be sufficiently distinct to warrant a provisional separate category in the REAL classification. This condition is probably what haematologists know as splenic lymphoma with villous lymphocytes.

2 NODAL. These cases are usually associated with disease elsewhere, e.g. MALTomas, and represent nodal spread. Occasionally the disease is restricted to lymph nodes with or without bone marrow involvement.

Histopathology of the bone marrow
Marginal zone lymphomas

Involvement of the bone marrow seems to be relatively uncommon so that descriptions in the literature are of individual cases rather than series. The commonest pattern is either the presence of central nodules or a patchy more diffuse infiltrate (Fig. 8.54).

Splenic lymphoma

Most of these cases have involvement of the bone marrow. The commonest pattern is similar to marginal zone lymphomas, i.e. with central nodules, though cases have been described which are entirely diffuse, some of which show plasmacytic differentiation with Dutcher bodies. Whether these latter cases have a relationship to immunocytoma is unclear (Fig. 8.55).

> **Immunophenotype:** IgM, IgD, CD19+, CD20+, CD22+, CD79+, CD5-, CD10-, CD23-

Diagnostic problems

These are uncommon lesions with the bone marrow usually being requested for staging purposes. It is doubtful that the histology of the bone marrow alone would allow a more precise diagnosis than low-grade B cell lymphoma.

> **Summary of key points**
> - Marginal zone lymphomas are mainly comprised of MALT lesions and their extensions into lymph nodes and other tissues.
> - MALT lesions rarely involve bone marrow unlike splenic lymphomas where marrow infiltration is common.
> - Splenic lymphoma is probably an entity distinct from marginal zone lymphoma.

Hairy cell leukaemia

Chapter   8.8

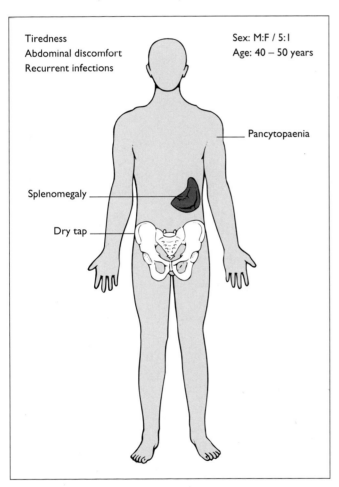

Tiredness
Abdominal discomfort
Recurrent infections

Sex: M:F / 5:1
Age: 40 – 50 years

Pancytopaenia

Splenomegaly

Dry tap

Fig 8.56 Major clinical features of a typical case of hairy cell leukaemia.

Introduction

Hairy cell leukaemia (HCL) was originally described as leukaemic reticuloendotheliosis. Its current terminology is inspired by the hair-like processes of the leukaemic cells seen by electron microscopic examination. Hairy cell leukaemia is a low-grade lymphoproliferative disorder of B lymphocytes which is now recognized as a distinct clinico-pathological entity.

Clinical features

The typical clinical picture is illustrated in Fig. 8.56.

Histopathology of the bone marrow

The cells are small (their nuclei being slightly larger than a resting lymphocyte) and lie spaced apart. The nuclei are oval or 'bean'-shaped, have one or two small inconspicuous nucleoli and are surrounded by a clear zone of cytoplasm (Fig. 8.57). The so-called hairs seen in smears and by electron microscopy are not apparent in conventional tissue sections (Fig. 8.58). Mitotic figures are rare.

A reticulin stain reveals fine fibrils distributed throughout the infiltrate, being present around almost every individual neoplastic cell. It is this extensive intercellular network of reticulin which is responsible for the 'dry tap' during aspiration biopsy. There is no fibrosis, i.e. collagen production (Fig. 8.59).

Patterns of involvement

The marrow is usually hypercellular. There are three main patterns of involvement by the neoplastic cells. All three patterns are often seen in the same specimen which is best appreciated by immuno-staining.

1 FOCAL INVOLVEMENT. This is the most common pattern with the neoplastic cells forming ill-defined groups interspersed with normal haematopoietic tissue. This type of distribution means that a single trephine biopsy may sample an unaffected area, missing the main foci of disease. If the diagnosis is considered, hairy cells may be demonstrated by immunostaining in more than 95% of cases. A useful reagent is antibody DBA.44 which, although incompletely

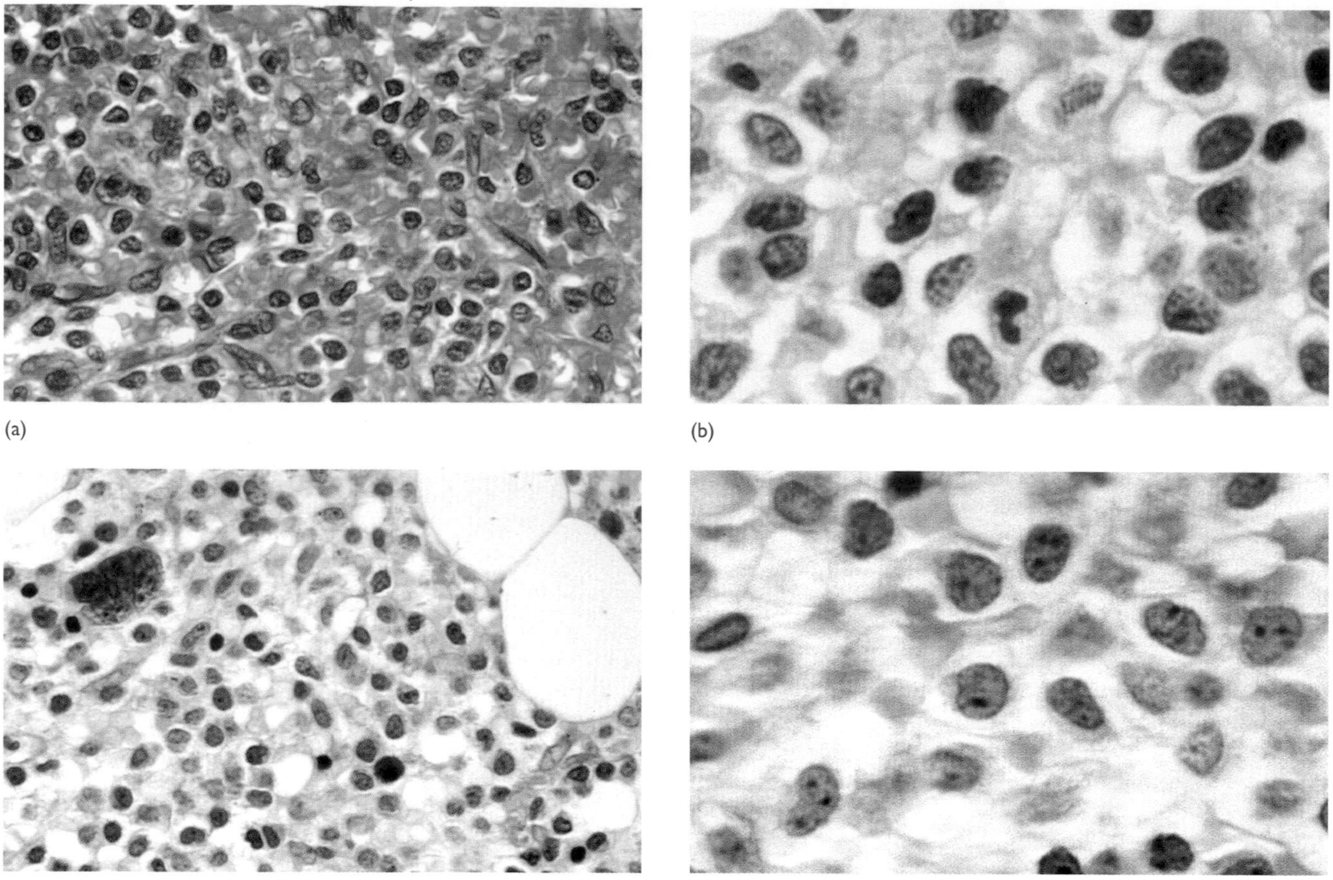

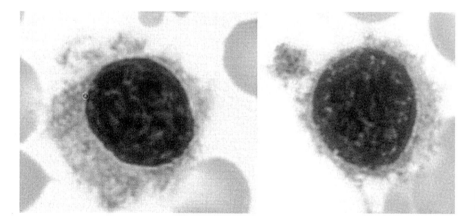

(a)

(b)

(c)

(d)

Fig 8.57 Typical case of hairy cell leukaemia in a bone marrow trephine. (a & b) H&E, medium and high power. (c & d) Giemsa, medium and high power.

Fig 8.58 Typical hairy cells in a bone marrow smear. Giemsa.

characterized, is a reliable marker of hairy cells in fixed specimens (Fig. 8.60).

2 DIFFUSE INVOLVEMENT. The hairy cells are dispersed throughout the marrow. This may range from a sparse infiltrate, easily overlooked, to virtual replacement of the marrow (Fig. 8.61).

3 INTERSTITIAL INVOLVEMENT. This is less common and refers to the presence of hairy cells lying amongst fat spaces in a hypoplastic marrow. In the absence of clinical suspicion they may be overlooked and a misdiagnosis of aplastic anaemia made (Fig. 8.62).

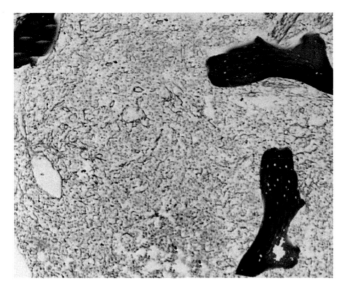

Fig 8.59 Reticulin stain showing the fine fibrillar meshwork in a bone marrow infiltrated by hairy cell leukaemia.

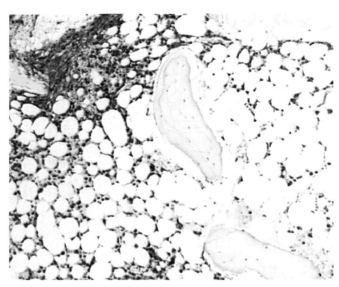

Fig 8.60 Focal area of hairy cell leukaemia highlighted by immunostaining for DBA.44 (arrow).

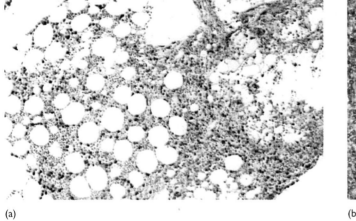

(a)

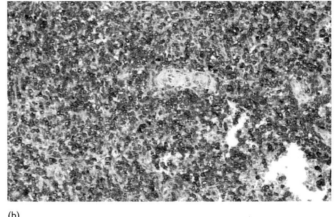

(b)

Fig 8.61 Diffuse infiltration, both sparse (a) and heavy (b), of bone marrow by hairy cells highlighted by immunostaining for (a) DBA.44, (b) CD79a.

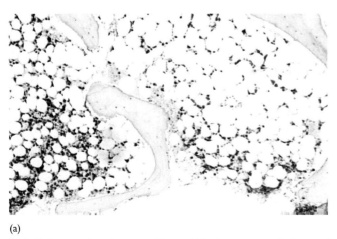

(a)

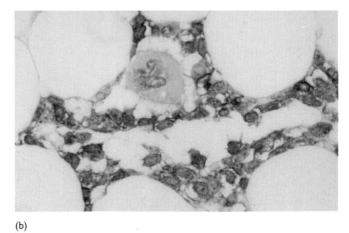

(b)

Fig 8.62 Interstitial involvement of hypocellular bone marrow by hairy cells. (a & b) Low and high power immunostaining for DBA.44.

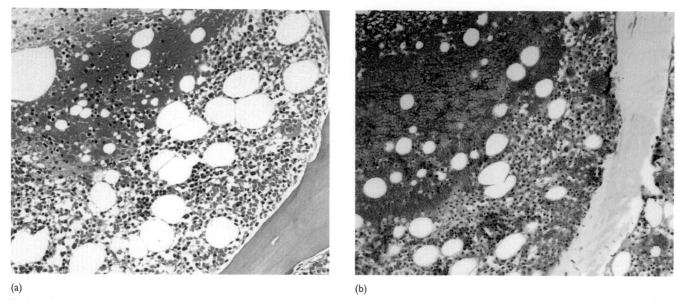

(a)   (b)

Fig 8.63 'Blood lakes' in hairy cell leukaemia. (a) H&E. (b) Immunostain for red cell glycophorin C.

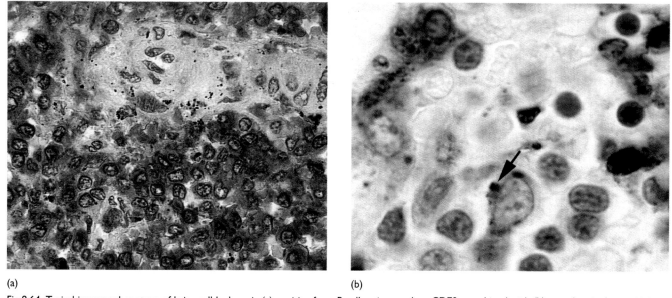

(a)   (b)

Fig 8.64 Typical immunophenotype of hairy cell leukaemia (a) positive for a B cell antigen such as CD79a combined with (b) cytoplasmic dot-positivity for CD68 (arrow). Positive staining for DBA.44 as illustrated earlier is also helpful.

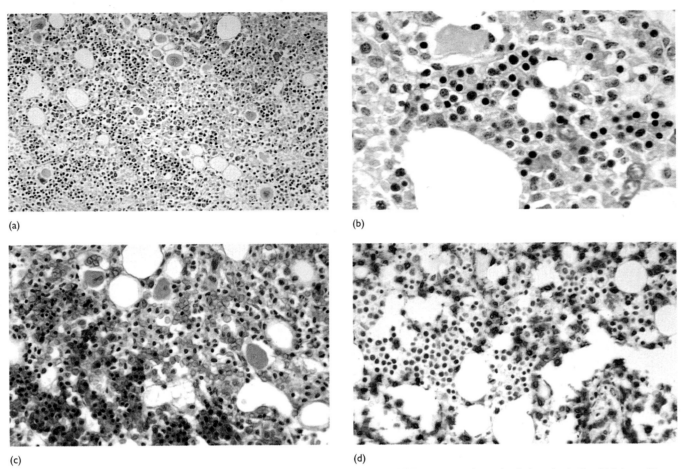

(a)

(b)

(c)

(d)

Fig 8.65 Hypercellular bone marrow with marked erythroid hyperplasia. (a & b) Giemsa. (c) Immunostain for red cell glycophorin C, which is masking the underlying infiltrate of hairy cell leukaemia. (d) Immunostain for B cell antigen, CD79a.

A useful diagnostic feature is that low-power observation of the involved trephine biopsy will often show focal areas of haemorrhage within the marrow. These are equivalent to the 'blood lakes' seen in sections of spleen involved by HCL (Fig. 8.63). Hairy cells are unique B cells which co-express many histiocytic antigens — a combination which is virtually diagnostic. For the fixed embedded trephine, positivity with the B cell antigens CD79a and CD20, combined with staining for CD68 and DBA.44, are a great assistance in establishing the diagnosis (Fig. 8.64).

Diagnostic problems

Differential diagnosis
In some cases of HCL the non-neoplastic marrow may show marked hyperplastic or even myelodysplastic features. If the hairy cell infiltrate is overlooked a misdiagnosis may be made (Fig. 8.65).

On occasion, other infiltrates may mimic hairy cell leukaemia, e.g. mesenchymal chondroblastoma[1] and systemic mast cell disease.[2]

Assessing extent of marrow involvement
The extent of marrow involvement by hairy cells is often requested by clinicians as it allows an estimation to be made of the tumour load response to treatment. Complex semi-quantitative procedures have been described in the literature but have not been widely adopted by pathologists. At the present time a reasonable compromise would seem to be a low-power estimate of percentage marrow involved based on immunostaining for hairy cells.

Assessing remission
Many patients with hairy cell leukaemia in clinical remission show small numbers of hairy cells in their marrows, especially after immunocytochemical examination. The significance and clinical

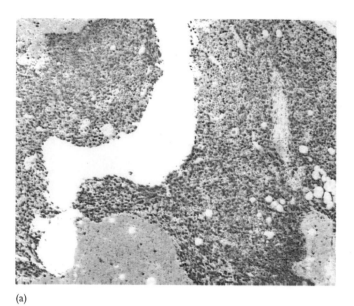

(a)

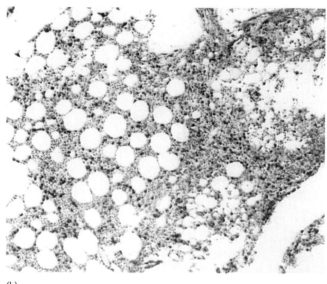

(b)

Fig 8.66 Bone marrow in 'remission' after treatment for hairy cell leukaemia still contains an infiltrate when immunostained for DBA.44. (a) Pretreatment. (b) Post-treatment.

relevance of such residual disease remains unclear. This has led some authorities to allow the marrow to contain small numbers of hairy cells and still qualify as complete remission (Fig. 8.66).[3]

Summary of key points
- Marrow involvement by hairy cells may be subtle.
- Characteristic histological features include:
  bean-shaped nuclei
  spaced-apart distribution
  delicate intercellular reticulin
  interstitial haemorrhage.
- Immunocytochemistry is of value, particularly in cases displaying subtle forms of marrow involvement.

References
1 Yam LT, Phyliky RL, Li C-Y. Benign and neoplastic disorders simulating Hairy cell leukaemia. *Seminars in Oncology* 1984; **11**: 353–361.
2 Webb TA, Li C-Y, Yam LT. Systemic mast cell disease; a clinical and haematopathologic study of 26 cases. *Cancer* 1982; **49**: 927–938.
3 Naeim F, Jacobs AD. Bone marrow changes in patients with hairy cell leukaemia treated by recombinant alpha-interferon. *Human Pathol* 1985; **16**: 1200–1205.

Multiple myeloma

Chapter 8.9

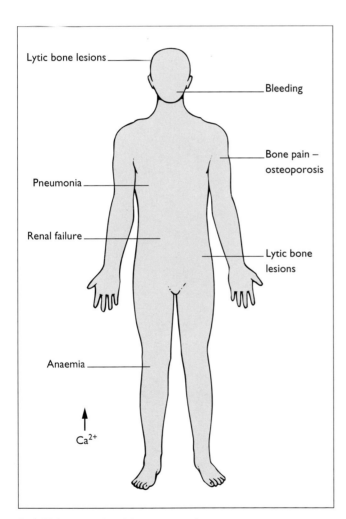

Fig 8.67 Common clinical features in myeloma.

Introduction

Multiple myeloma is a clinical entity caused by a malignant mono-clonal proliferation of plasma cells within the bone marrow. It is characterized by

(a) increased numbers of clonal plasma cells within the bone marrow (> 10% of the nucleated cell population),

(b) lytic bone lesions and

(c) the presence of an M (or paraprotein) band identified electrophoretically in serum or urine.

At least two of these three components must be present before a diagnosis of myeloma can be made.

Clinical features

The commonest clinical features associated with myeloma are illustrated in Fig. 8.67.

The clinical course is typically a cycle of remission following chemotherapy with eventual relapse into high-grade disease which is resistant to further chemotherapy. An indolent form, known as smouldering myeloma, has been described.[1]

Histopathology of the bone marrow

The marrow is typically hypercellular (Fig. 8.68). The normal haematopoietic elements still remain but are overrun by neoplastic

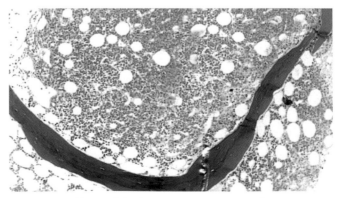

Fig 8.68 Typical hypercellular bone marrow in myeloma. Giemsa.

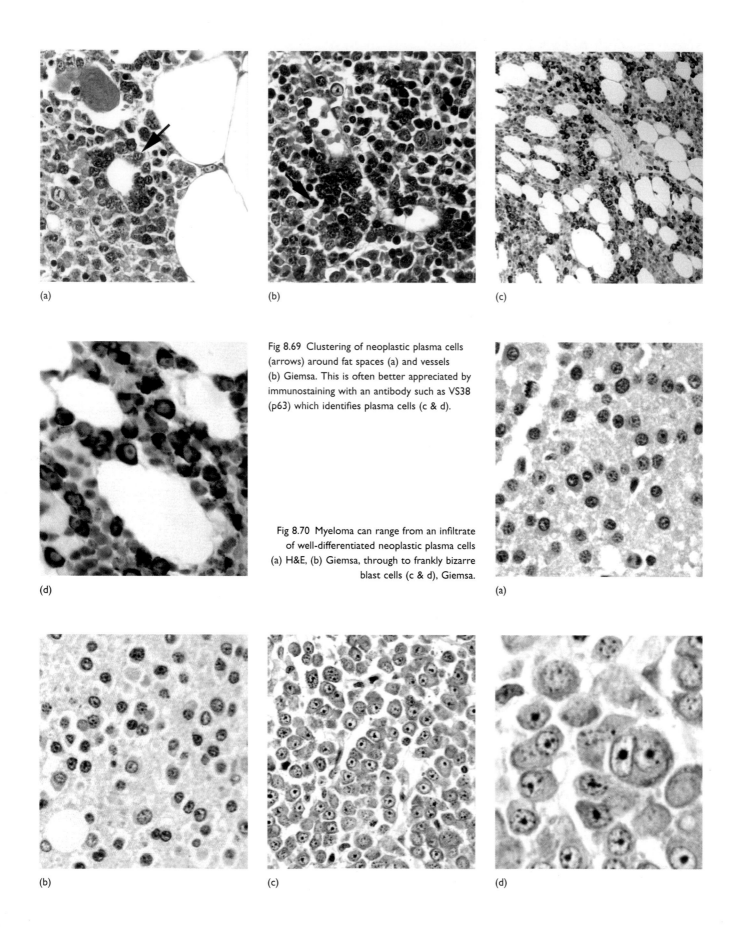

(a)

(b)

(c)

Fig 8.69 Clustering of neoplastic plasma cells (arrows) around fat spaces (a) and vessels (b) Giemsa. This is often better appreciated by immunostaining with an antibody such as VS38 (p63) which identifies plasma cells (c & d).

(d)

Fig 8.70 Myeloma can range from an infiltrate of well-differentiated neoplastic plasma cells (a) H&E, (b) Giemsa, through to frankly bizarre blast cells (c & d), Giemsa.

(a)

(b)

(c)

(d)

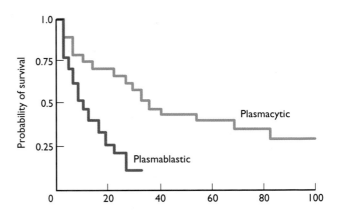

Histologic groups	Main subtype	Survival (months)
Plasmacytic		
Marshalko		46
Small round		24
Small notched		19
Polymorphous		16
Plasmablastic		9

Fig 8.71 Range of differentiation of neoplastic plasma cells in myeloma and their relationship to survival.

Table 8.3 A comparison of the histological features of reactive plasmacytosis and multiple myeloma.

Reactive plasmacytosis	Multiple myeloma
Plasma cells usually constitute < 25% of cells	Plasma cells usually constitute > 25% of cells
Majority are mature plasma cells	Greater variation in size
Nucleoli only present in a few plasma cells	Nucleoli often present
Collections, i.e. nodules or sheets of plasma cells, never seen	Often present in large homogeneous groups
Occasional bi-nucleated forms and less mature forms	Plasmablast forms (prominent central nucleoli)
Single layer around capillaries	Several cells deep around capillaries, diffusely distributed amongst fat cells, groups or sheets of plasma cells

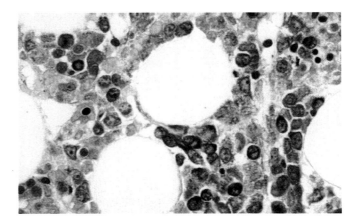

Fig 8.72 Reactive plasmacytosis in HIV infection.

plasma cells. These are usually distributed throughout the marrow space and tend to be organized in irregular clusters or in peri-vascular multilayers (Fig. 8.69).

Abnormal forms (bi- or multi-nucleate and blast cells) are typically present but the neoplastic cells may be so well-differentiated as to be indistinguishable from normal reactive plasma cells (Fig. 8.70). Patient survival can be related to the plasma cell morphology (Fig. 8.71).[2]

The histological features which may be used to distinguish reactive plasmacytosis from multiple myeloma are described in Table 8.3.

None of these criteria is absolute. Some conditions produce a marked plasmacytosis which is purely reactive in nature, e.g. HIV infection and hepatitis (Fig. 8 72).

The only certain means of separating the two conditions is by demonstrating monoclonality. This is most easily done immuno-

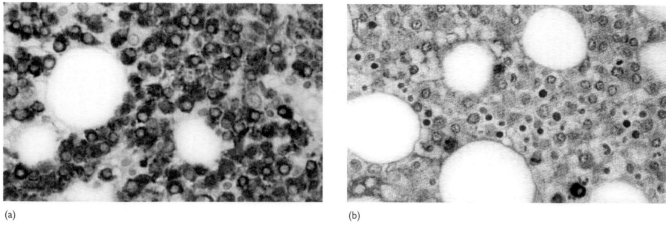

(a)   (b)

Fig 8.73 Light chain restriction in myeloma. Lambda-positive myeloma cells (a) greatly outnumber a few remaining benign kappa-positive cells (b).

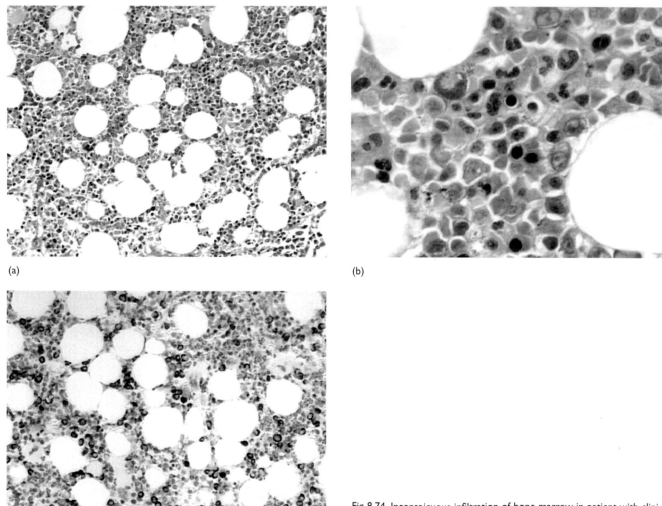

(a)   (b)

(c)

Fig 8.74 Inconspicuous infiltration of bone marrow in patient with clinical myeloma. (a & b) Giemsa. (c) Immunostain for VS38. Light chain immunostaining demonstrated monoclonality.

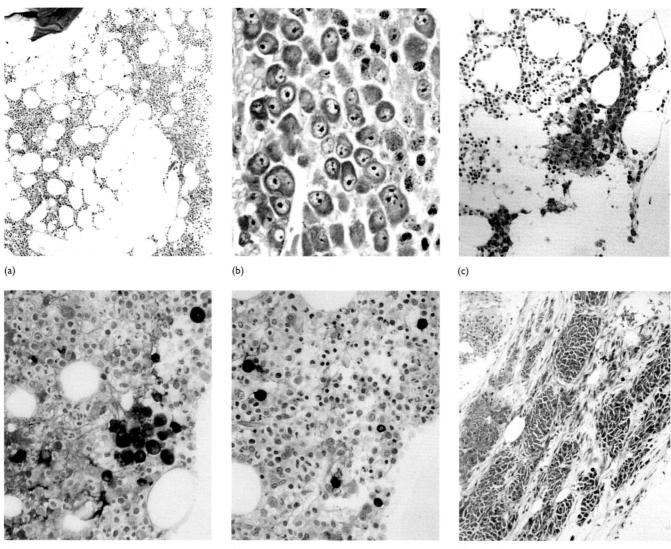

(a)

(b)

(c)

(d)

(e)

Fig 8.75 Focal infiltration of myeloma. (a & b) Giemsa. (c) VS38 immunostain for plasma cells. (d) Lambda and (e) kappa light chain immunostains.

Fig 8.76 Cohesive clumps of myeloma cells mimicking metastatic carcinoma.

histochemically by showing the presence of light chain restriction. Reactive plasma cells will have a ratio of about two kappa-positive cells to every lambda-positive cell. In contrast, myeloma cells will all belong to the same clone and secrete only one type of light chain. There are always some reactive plasma cells mixed in with the myeloma cells so in practice monoclonality is identified by a ratio outside the normal 2:1. Typically a ratio of 10:1 of kappa to lambda or 5:1 if lambda is the dominant type provides evidence for the neoplastic nature of the plasma cells (Fig. 8.73).

On a practical note, one should be reluctant to accept immunostaining as reliable if all the plasma cells are negative for one of the light chains (there should be a few positive reactive plasma cells), since this is more likely to indicate technical failure rather than an exclusive type of light chain production.

Less common appearances
(a) Myeloma cells can be inconspicuous when they are present in small numbers and infiltrate the marrow diffusely without any clustering (Fig. 8.74).
(b) The infiltration may be focal and not aspirated (Fig. 8.75).
(c) Myeloma cells may form cohesive groups which can be mistaken for metastatic disease such as breast cancer (Fig. 8.76).

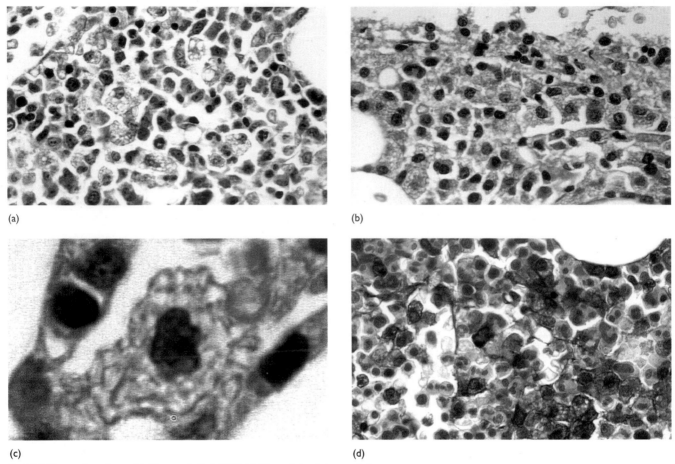

Fig 8.77 Mott cell myeloma. (a) Giemsa. (b & c) H&E. (d) Kappa light chain restriction.

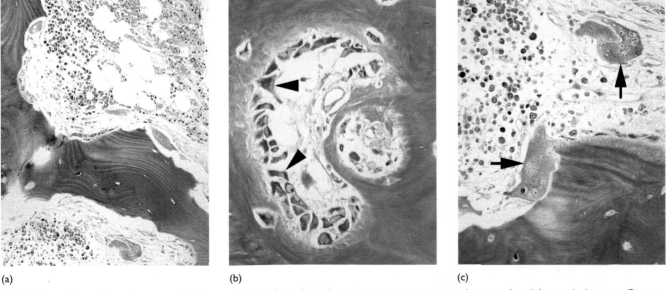

Fig 8.78 Bone changes in myeloma caused by increased osteoblastic (arrowheads) and osteoclastic (arrows) activity. (a – c) Low to high power. Giemsa.

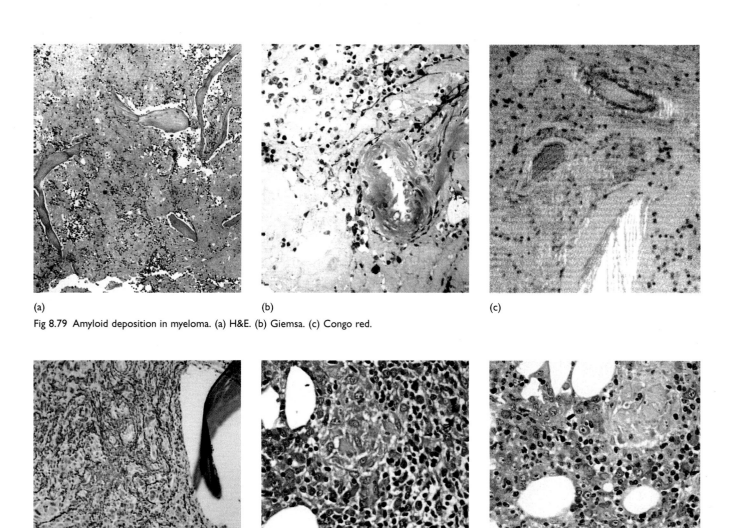

Fig 8.79 Amyloid deposition in myeloma. (a) H&E. (b) Giemsa. (c) Congo red.

(a)

(b)

(c)

Fig 8.80 Increased reticulin staining in a case of myeloma.

(a)

(b)

Fig 8.81 Granuloma formation associated with myeloma. (a) H&E. (b) Giemsa.

(d) The myeloma cells may have a vacuolated cytoplasm (Mott cells) which can be misidentified as histiocytes or mucus-producing cells (Fig. 8.77).

In all of these situations the most valuable diagnostic aid is light chain immunostaining.

Other features occasionally seen in association with myeloma

(a) Destruction of the bone by osteoclasts causing the characteristic lytic lesions in myeloma. The neoplastic plasma cells themselves do not resorb bone (Fig. 8.78).

(b) The secretion of light chains by the myeloma cells can lead to the deposition of amyloid within the marrow (Fig. 8.79).

(c) About 10% of myeloma cases will have increased reticulin staining and hence a trephine biopsy is more likely to be diagnostic than an aspirate (Fig. 8.80).

(d) The presence of sarcoid-like granulomas occurs occasionally in myeloma. Its significance is unclear (Fig. 8.81).[3]

(e) Multiple reactive lymphoid aggregates (> three per low-power field) may be found in a minority of cases and are said to be associated with fewer lytic bone lesions.[4]

(f) Other malignancies such as chronic myeloproliferative disorders and acute leukaemias may be found coexisting with myeloma in the marrow.

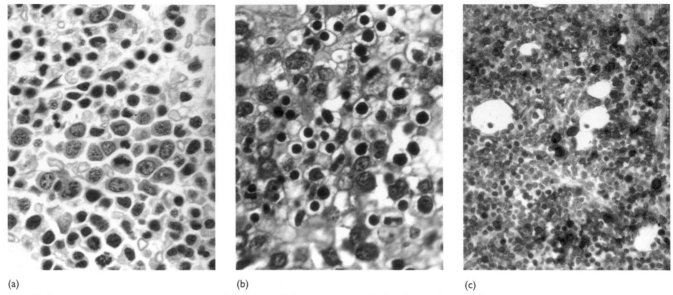

(a)   (b)   (c)

Fig 8.82 Erythroblasts resemble plasmablasts by H&E staining (a) but are more easily identified by Giemsa (b) or immunostaining for red cell antigens such as glycophorin C (c).

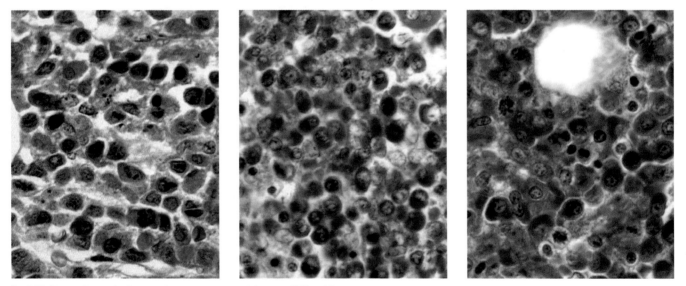

Fig 8.83 Promyelocytic leukaemia showing prominent 'plasma cell'-like differentiation.

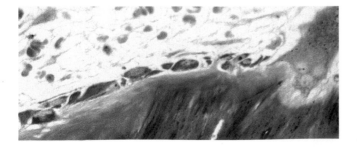

Fig 8.84 Osteoblasts may look remarkably like plasma cells but are readily identified by their paratrabecular location.

Diagnostic problems

What is the significance of a low number of monoclonal plasma cells in a marrow?

The detection of a neoplastic population of plasma cells in a marrow, where the full criteria for multiple myeloma are not met, probably reflects our ability to detect the disease at an earlier stage in its development than had been possible before the introduction of immunohistochemical techniques. A small number of asymptomatic individuals (usually elderly) in the population have a monoclonal band in their serum. This is not of light chain type, as is usually the case in myeloma, but is IgG or IgM. The neoplastic clone secreting this paraprotein is usually too small to detect in bone marrow biopsies. These cases have been called monoclonal gammopathy of uncertain significance (MGUS) or benign paraproteinemia. Whilst some cases (about 30% over a 10-year period) progress to myelomatosis the majority appear to remain healthy. Thus detection of a plasma cell monoclone in the marrow is not *per se* definite evidence of incipient myeloma. Obviously such individuals will require careful monitoring.

What other cells resemble plasma cells?

I ERYTHROBLASTS

Plasmablasts may resemble erythroblasts, since both cell types possess a paranuclear hof. This is especially apparent in H&E-stained sections whereas Giemsa staining reveals a delicate blue in erythroid cytoplasm contrasting with the lilac hue of the plasmablast (Fig. 8.82). In addition, the plasmablast has a single nucleolus whilst the erythroblast usually has more than one. Groups of erythroblasts are often found in association with more mature, and therefore more readily identified, elements such as normoblasts. Unequivocal evidence of a cell's nature is provided by immunohistochemistry for erythroid and lymphoid markers.

2 PROMYELOCYTES

The promyelocytes of acute promyelocytic leukaemia may resemble plasma cells as their nucleus is eccentrically placed and their cytoplasm plentiful. The chromatin pattern is quite different since the promyelocyte's nucleus is densely staining and lacks the plasma cell's 'clock face' nucleus or the plasmablast's prominent solitary nucleolus. Immunohistochemistry will easily resolve those cases where doubt remains (Fig. 8.83).

3 OSTEOBLASTS

Although it is unlikely to be a source of diagnostic difficulty, it should be remembered that osteoblasts morphologically resemble plasma cells. Their distinctive paratrabecular distribution readily identifies their true nature (Fig. 8.84).

Summary of key points
- Immunohistochemistry is invaluable in separating reactive plasmacytosis from multiple myeloma and in identifying cases of 'early' myeloma where the number of plasma cells is low.
- The degree of plasma cell differentiation and pattern of marrow involvement may relate to prognosis.
- Whilst most cases of myeloma are diagnostically straightforward a few cases will involve the marrow more subtly. Careful inspection of the marrow section and the use of immunocytochemistry will reveal them.

References
1 Kyle RA, Greipp PR. Smoldering multiple myeloma. *New England J Med* 1980; **302**: 1347–1349.
2 Bartl R, Frisch B. Bone marrow histology in multiple myeloma: prognostic relevance of histologic characteristics. *Haematological reviews* 1989; **3**: 87–108.
3 Falini B, Tabilio A, Veelardi A, Cernetti C, Aversa F, Martelli MF. Multiple myeloma with a sarcoidosis-like reaction. *Scand J Haematol* 1982; **29**: 211–216.
4 Aghai E, Avni G, Lurie M, Quitt M, Hornstein L, Froom P. Bone marrow biopsy in multiple myeloma: a clinical pathological study. *Isr J Med Sci* 1988; **24**: 298–301.

Diffuse large B cell lymphoma

Chapter 8.10

General features 111
Histopathology of the bone marrow 112
Diagnostic problems 114
Summary of key points 114

General features

Within the REAL classification, this entity encompasses a number of conditions described by Kiel and other groups. These include centroblastic, immunoblastic and T-cell-rich B cell lymphoma. The REAL group has suggested at least provisionally incorporating all of these lesions as one entity since even experienced pathologists have great difficulty in recognizing those subdivisions described to date (Fig. 8.85).

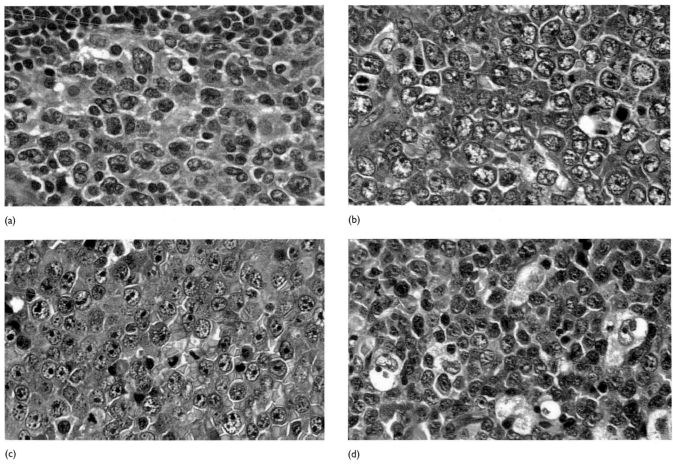

(a)

(b)

(c)

(d)

Fig 8.85 Four different large B cell lymphomas illustrating the cellular heterogeneity of this category.

111

Large cell lymphomas with an anaplastic morphology are currently included in this category and not as anaplastic large cell lymphomas. A further justification for this grouping is that at present there is no evidence to suggest that the treatment or prognosis of any of these conditions differs (Fig. 8.86).

Large cell lymphomas constitute about 40% of adult NHL. Most patients are over 40 years old and present with rapidly enlarging lymph nodes although a substantial minority of cases will be extranodal. It is an aggressive but potentially curable condition.

Histopathology of the bone marrow

The neoplastic cells have large vesicular nuclei, prominent nucleoli, basophilic cytoplasm and easily found mitotic figures. There is a variability in the morphology of these large cells which gave rise to their description as separate categories in other classifications. In practice these lymphomas usually have a heterogeneous cell population which has made for high intra- and inter-observer error in classification (Fig. 8.87).

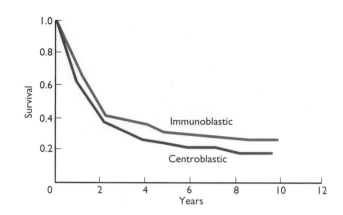

Fig 8.86 Survival curve of centroblastic and immunoblastic lymphomas diagnosed by Kiel criteria.

Immunophenotype: surface Ig+/-, CD19+, CD20+ CD22+, CD79a+, CD10-/+, CD5-/+, CD45+/-

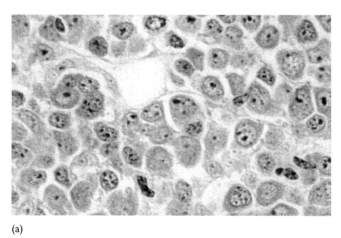

(a)

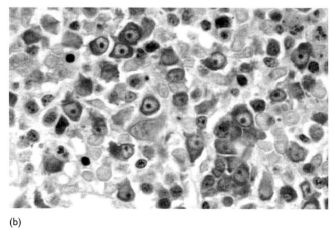

(b)

Fig 8.87 Two typical examples of large cell lymphoma in the bone marrow. Note the high degree of cellular heterogeneity. Giemsa.

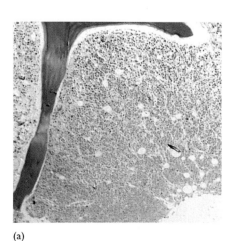

(a)

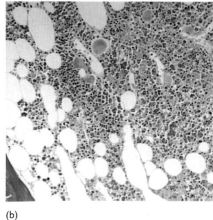

(b)

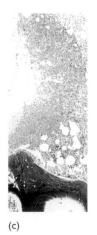

(c)

Fig 8.88 Different patterns of involvement of the bone marrow by large cell lymphoma. Giemsa.

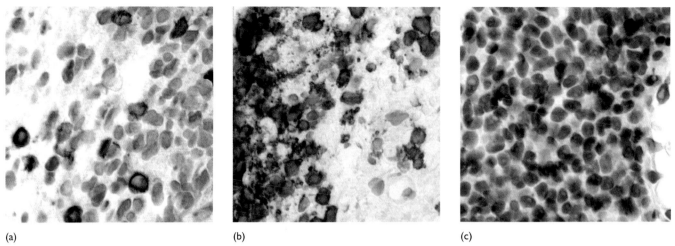

(a)   (b)   (c)

Fig 8.89 T-cell-rich large B cell lymphoma in the bone marrow. (a) CD79 (B cell). (b) CD3 (T cell). (c) Ki67 (proliferation marker).

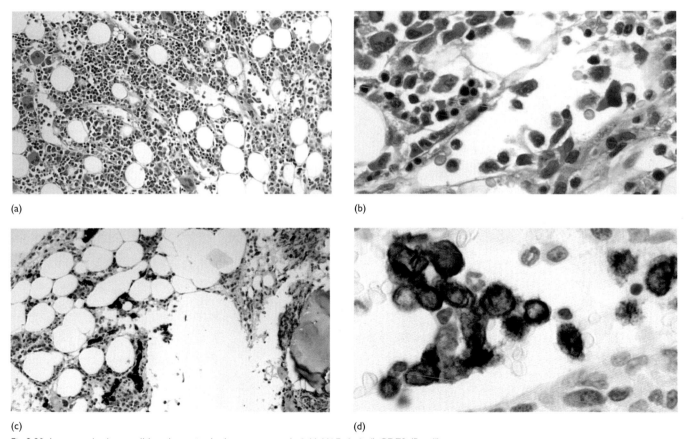

(a)

(b)

(c)

(d)

Fig 8.90 Intravascular large cell lymphoma in the bone marrow. (a & b) H&E. (c & d) CD79 (B cell).

When present, involvement of bone marrow is usually obvious but without any particular histological pattern (Fig. 8.88).

Occasionally large B cell lymphomas consist only of scattered malignant cells with a florid T cell reaction known as T-cell-rich B cell lymphomas (Fig. 8.89).

A rare variant easily missed on morphology alone is the intravascular large cell lymphoma previously known as 'malignant angioendotheliosis' (Fig. 8.90).

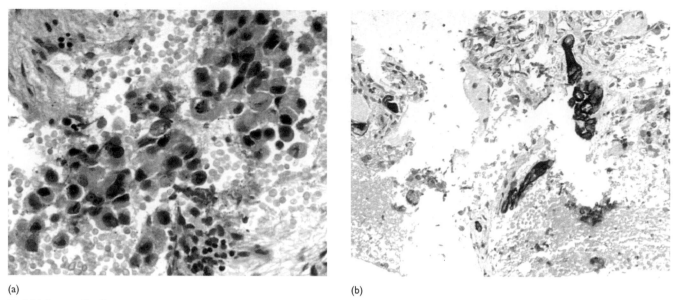

(a)

(b)

Fig 8.91 Large cell infiltrate in bone marrow (a: H&E) initially thought to be lymphoma but shown to be secondary carcinoma by immunostaining. (b) Cytokeratin immunostain.

Antibody	Large cell anaplastic morphology*	Other large cell	Carcinoma
CD45	-/+	+	-
CD30	+/-	-/+	-
CD20	+	+	-
CD3	-	-	-
anti-cytokeratins	-	-	+
EMA	-/+	-	+/-
*These B cell cases are classified as large cell lymphomas not anaplastic lymphomas in the REAL scheme.			

Table 8.4 Differential diagnosis of anaplastic lymphomas.

Diagnostic problems

Large B cell lymphoma vs. anaplastic carcinoma

It is important to make the distinction between these two groups since the treatment regimes differ and a cure is more likely in the lymphoma group if appropriate treatment is given. Distinction is possible immunohistochemically (Fig. 8.91).

In those cases with an anaplastic large cell morphology, the resemblance to metastatic carcinoma may be strong. The antibodies shown in Table 8.4 will help in distinguishing between these groups.

Summary of key points
- Diffuse large B cell lymphomas consist of several morphological types.
- They are clinically aggressive but potentially curable.
- Distinction must be made from anaplastic carcinoma.

Burkitt's lymphoma

General features

This lymphoma occurs in two different settings although the histological appearances are identical. The African (endemic) form is the commonest childhood (4–7 years) malignancy in parts of equatorial Africa and in New Guinea. The lymphoma tends to involve the jaw, either mandible or maxilla, and may extend up into the orbit. Other organs are commonly involved, e.g. ovary, testes, liver, retroperitoneum, breast and gastrointestinal tract. It is associated with Epstein–Barr virus (EBV) and involves a chromosomal translocation commonly t(8;14).

The non-African (non-endemic) form is a rare lymphoma and occurs over a wider age range with many adult cases, often those with an immunodeficiency, and involves the gastrointestinal tract (particularly the terminal ileum), ovaries and kidneys. Lymph node involvement is less frequently seen than in most other lymphomas. EBV is associated with a minority of these cases, usually those with immunodeficiency.

The genetic features suggest that the endemic form is a neoplasm involving an early B cell whilst the non-endemic form arises from a B cell at a later stage of development.

The lymphoma is highly aggressive, having the fastest doubling time of any known human neoplasm, although it is potentially curable.

Histopathology of the bone marrow

The marrow is involved in about 20% of non-endemic cases.

The neoplastic cell has the same appearance in both forms of the disease. It is a medium-sized blast cell with a moderate amount of basophilic cytoplasm and a regular oval or round nucleus containing 2–5 small nucleoli (Fig. 8.92). Mitotic figures are numerous, although the 'starry sky' appearance seen in other organs is not a feature (Fig. 8.93). Frank necrosis may be seen, particularly following chemotherapy. The marrow is usually hypercellular although interstitial, nodular and diffuse patterns of infiltration may occur (Fig. 8.94).

> **Immunophenotype**: SlgM+, CD19+, CD20+, CD22+, CD79a+, CD10+, CD5- ,CD23- ,TdT-

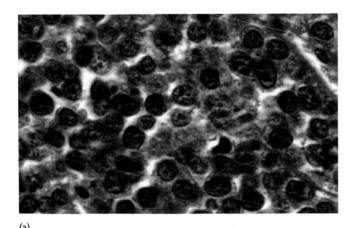

(a)

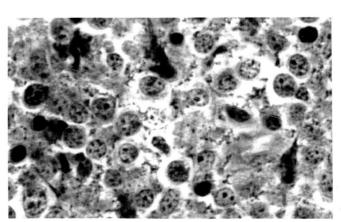

(b)

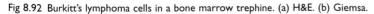

Fig 8.92 Burkitt's lymphoma cells in a bone marrow trephine. (a) H&E. (b) Giemsa.

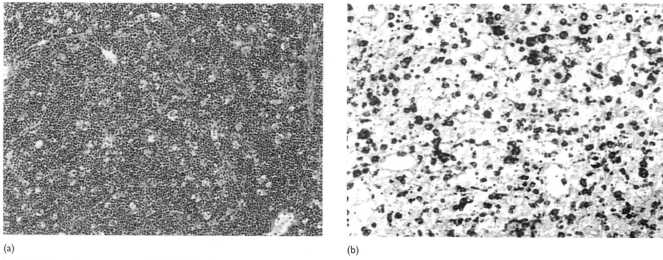

(a)   (b)

Fig 8.93 Starry sky appearance of Burkitt's lymphoma as seen in lymph nodes is uncommon in bone marrow sections. (a) H&E (ovary). (b) CD68 immunostain for macrophages.

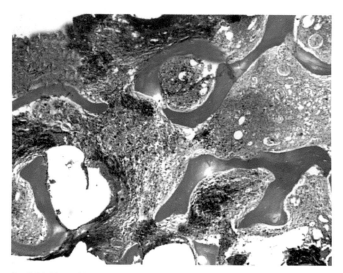

Fig 8.94 Typical low power picture of Burkitt's lymphoma in a bone marrow trephine.

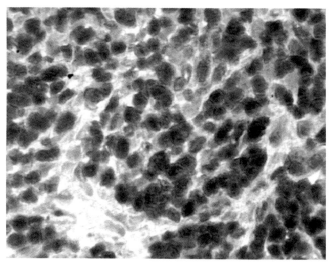

Fig 8.95 Virtually all nuclei are immunostained for Ki67 in Burkitt's lymphoma.

Diagnostic problems
Burkitt's vs. lymphoblastic lymphoma

Similarities exist between these two high-grade lymphomas; indeed for some time the Kiel classification treated Burkitt's lymphoma as a sub-type of lymphoblastic lymphoma. Careful evaluation of the nuclear morphology, in particular the multiple nucleoli seen in Burkitt's, is useful in separating the two entities. This is not always as easy as some texts make out. It is often worth examining the figures in such texts and on putting one's thumb over the starry sky macrophage seeing if a difference can be perceived. Assessment of proliferation with antibodies such as Ki67 may be helpful since in Burkitt's lymphoma all (or nearly all!) of the viable tumour cells will be positive (Fig. 8.95). In addition Burkitt's lymphoma cells do not express TdT.

Burkitt's vs. anaplastic carcinoma

The relatively abundant cytoplasm of the lymphoma cells and their tendency to form 'cohesive' clumps may impart an impression of carcinoma. Immunohistochemistry for lymphoid and epithelial markers will easily distinguish between the two diseases.

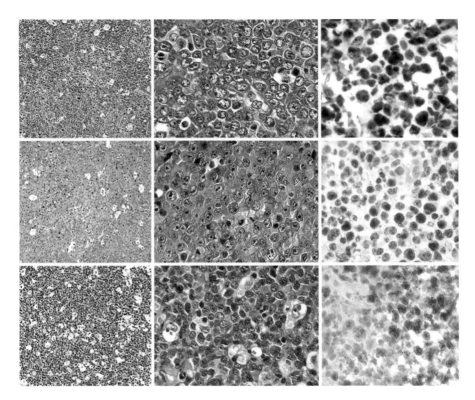

Fig 8.96 Three separate cases of Burkitt-like NHL (as identified by some members of the International Lymphoma Study Group) showing left to right low and high power and an immunostain for Ki67 illustrating the range of cases which may be given this categorization.

Burkitt's vs. large cell lymphoma

Occasional cases arise where it is difficult to distinguish between these two conditions. In these cases the neoplastic cells are more pleomorphic and larger than typical Burkitt's lymphoma cell, with larger numbers of nucleoli. These cases have been provisionally categorized in the REAL classification as high-grade B cell lymphoma, Burkitt-like. It is particularly frequently recognized by US pathologists where it is also known as non-Burkitt's lymphoma (Fig. 8.96).

These rare cases tend to involve adults and present with node involvement. Immunohistochemically they usually differ from typical Burkitt's by being CD10 negative. Once again, Ki67 staining will be most helpful since only Burkitt's lymphoma will have practically all cell nuclei labelled.

Summary of key points
- Two forms exist: an endemic and a non-endemic. Although histologically identical, they have different clinical presentations.
- Very high proliferation rate as demonstrated by antibodies, e.g. Ki67 or mib-1.
- Immunohistochemistry will distinguish between anaplastic carcinoma and lymphoblastic lymphoma.

Large granular lymphocyte (LGL) leukaemia

General features

This is an uncommon condition also described as CD8 lymphocytosis with neutropenia or Tγ lymphoproliferative disease. The peripheral blood lymphocytosis is composed of cells with round or oval nuclei with moderately condensed chromatin and rare nucleoli, eccentrically placed in abundant pale blue cytoplasm with azurophilic granules (Fig. 8.97).

There are two major lineages, one being T cell and the other having a natural killer (NK) cell phenotype. Patients with the T cell phenotype show clonal rearrangement of the T cell receptor genes whereas clonality has not been proven in the NK cell cases. T cell cases are predominantly a disease of late middle age and are associated with recurrent bacterial infections (a consequence of the invariable neutropenia). About 30% of patients have rheumatoid arthritis and Felty's or a Felty's-like syndrome. The clinical course is usually indolent.

NK cell cases are usually younger with more severe clinical symptoms of anaemia and thrombocytopaenia and more widespread tissue infiltration. Clonal cytogenetic abnormalities associated with EB virus infection have been reported in a number of clinically aggressive cases from Japan.

Although debate continues whether LGL proliferations are reactive or neoplastic it is being progressively accepted as a leukaemia based on the observations of clonality and tissue invasion by LGLs of marrow, spleen and liver.

Histopathology of the bone marrow

Bone marrow infiltration is usually sparse, with mild to moderate lymphocytosis as well as focal nodules composed of both B and T cells. A diagnosis is unlikely on the trephine alone which is easily misinterpreted as a B cell lymphoma (Fig. 8.98).

The key to the diagnosis is the peripheral blood smear which can be confirmed by splenic histology if the spleen is removed (Fig. 8.99). There may be a myeloid maturation arrest or erythroid hypoplasia.

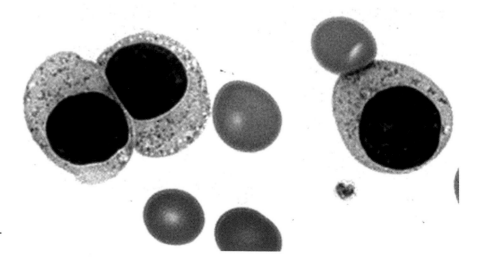

Fig. 8.97 The cytology of large granular lymphocytes in peripheral blood.

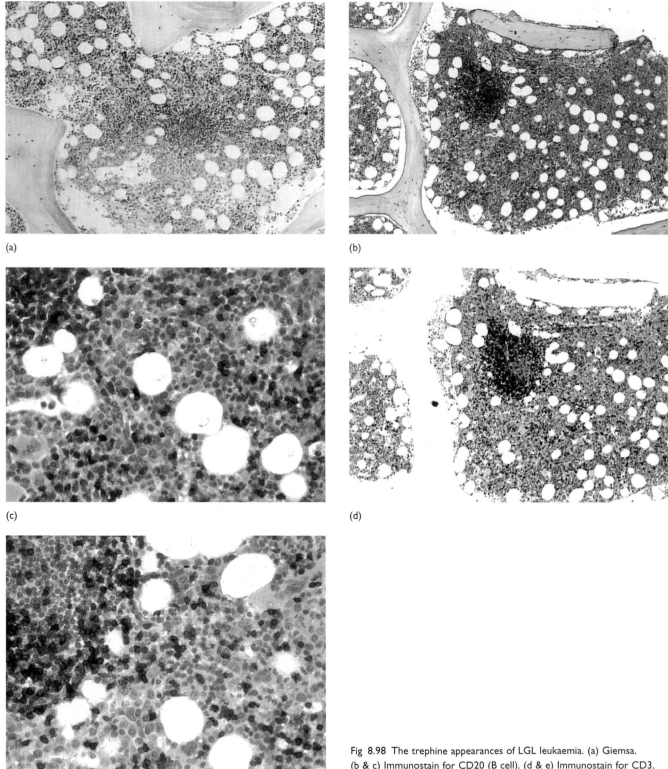

(a)

(b)

(c)

(d)

(e)

Fig 8.98 The trephine appearances of LGL leukaemia. (a) Giemsa.
(b & c) Immunostain for CD20 (B cell). (d & e) Immunostain for CD3.

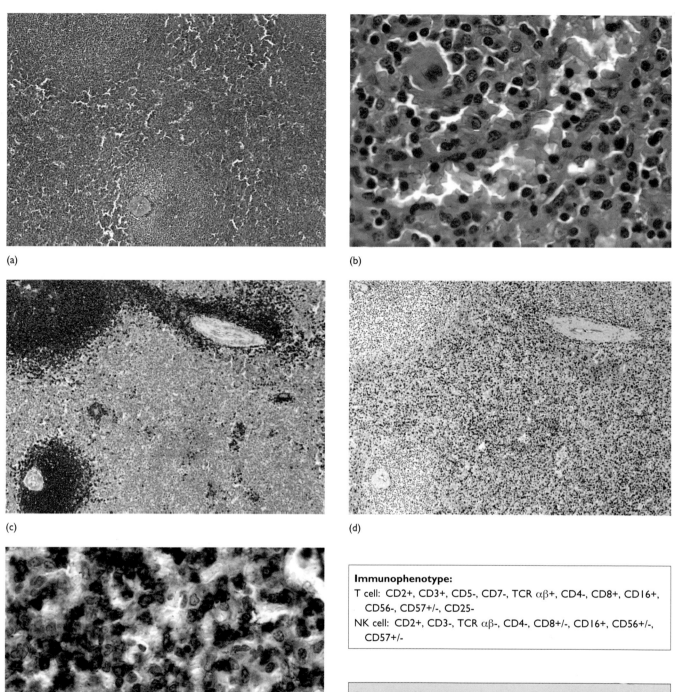

(a)

(b)

(c)

(d)

(e)

Immunophenotype:

T cell: CD2+, CD3+, CD5-, CD7-, TCR αβ+, CD4-, CD8+, CD16+, CD56-, CD57+/-, CD25-

NK cell: CD2+, CD3-, TCR αβ-, CD4-, CD8+/-, CD16+, CD56+/-, CD57+/-

Summary of key points

- LGL leukaemia has two types, T cell and NK cell.
- The clinical course is usually indolent apart from a subset of aggressive Asian NK cases.
- Marrow infiltration is subtle and may be misdiagnosed as B cell lymphoma.

Fig 8.99 The spleen in LGL leukaemia. (a & b) H&E. (c) CD20.
(d) CD3. (e) CD8.

Cutaneous T cell lymphoma

Chapter 8.13

General features

Most primary lymphomas of the skin are of two T cell types, mycosis fungoides or Sézary syndrome.

Mycosis fungoides more frequently affects middle-aged men and presents with single or multiple scaly skin lesions. The clinical progression is slow, often over 15 or 20 years, and the disease tends to remain localized to the skin although the lesions may become tumorous and ulcerate. Visceral and nodal involvement tend to occur late in the course of the disease.

Sézary syndrome can be viewed as the leukaemic counterpart of mycosis fungoides. It also has a cutaneous component but this tends to be much more extensive, existing as a pruritic generalized exfoliating erythroderma ('rouge homme'). Nodal involvement is common. The average life expectancy is 5 years.

Transformation to a large cell lymphoma, often of anaplastic large cell type, may occur as a terminal event in either form of primary cutaneous T cell lymphoma.

Histopathology of the bone marrow

The marrow is rarely involved, even in patients with advanced disease or Sézary syndrome. The neoplastic cell is usually of the T cell helper (CD4) type and morphologically is small with a convoluted (cerebriform) nucleus. Occasional larger cells may be present and these too have convoluted nuclei. There is no characteristic pattern of marrow involvement (Fig. 8.100).

> **Immunophenotype:** CD2+, CD3+, CD5+, CD7+(30%), CD4+, CD25-

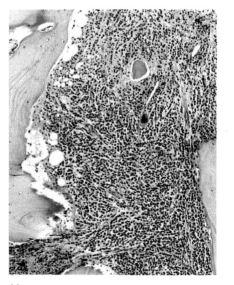

(a)

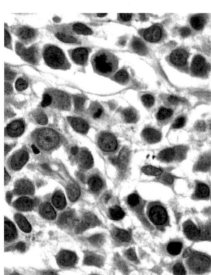

(b)

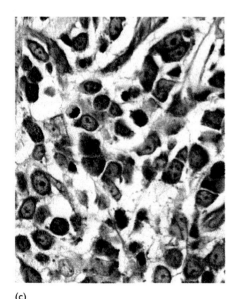

(c)

Fig 8.100 Large cell lymphoma infiltrating bone marrow as a terminal event in long-standing mycosis fungoides. (a & b) H&E. (c) Giemsa.

Diagnostic problems

The distinctive and readily observed clinical features of this condition and ease with which skin biopsies can be undertaken mean that diagnostic difficulties relating to marrow diagnosis are unlikely.

Summary of key points
- Primary cutaneous T cell lymphoma has two clinical forms.
- It usually is of T helper immunophenotype.
- The marrow is rarely involved.

Peripheral T cell lymphomas, unspecified

Chapter 8.14

General features

The REAL classification recognizes the difficulty faced by histopathologists in subclassifying T cell lymphomas and has created a category called 'peripheral T cell lymphomas, unspecified'. This category includes those cases which do not have distinct clinical syndromes that correspond to recognizable morphological subtypes. Whilst the Kiel classification recognizes as separate entities T-zone lymphoma, lymphoepithelioid cell lymphoma (Lennert's),

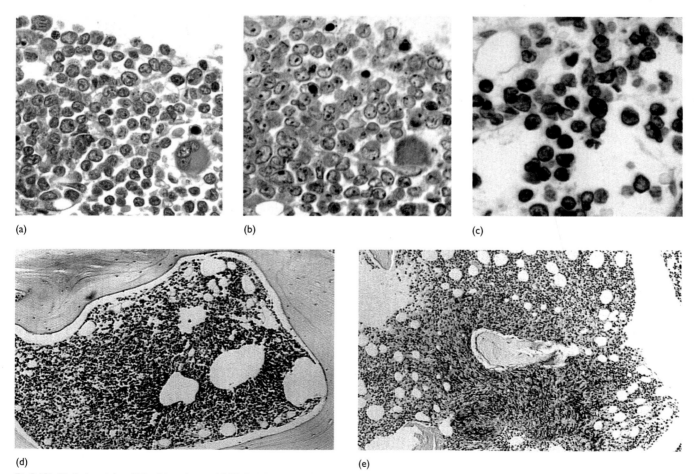

(a)

(b)

(c)

(d)

(e)

Fig 8.101 Typical peripheral T cell lymphoma. (a) H&E. (b) Giemsa. (c) Immunostain for CD3. Two different patterns of infiltration are shown by immunostaining for T cells (d & e).

T-immunoblastic and pleomorphic lymphoma, the REAL classification groups these diseases together under the heading of peripheral T cell lymphoma, unspecified.

The clinical features are varied. Most patients are adults with lymphadenopathy, skin (pruritis) and occasionally abdominal visceral involvement. Eosinophilia and a haemophagocytic syndrome may occur. The clinical course is usually aggressive and histological grade is less useful as a predictor of clinical behaviour than it is for B cell lymphomas.

Histopathology of the bone marrow

Given the unspecified nature of this entity it is not surprising that there are no unequivocal figures on marrow involvement. It would appear to be relatively common, i.e. up to 40% of cases. The pattern of infiltration is variable and can be interstitial, paratrabecular or both. The infiltrate is similar to that in the tissues being polymorphous with variable numbers of small, medium and large neoplastic atypical lymphoid cells admixed with eosinophils and histiocytes, some of which may be epithelioid. The neoplastic cells have irregular nuclei and some larger cells may resemble Reed–Sternberg cells (Fig. 8.101).

> **Immunophenotype:** CD3+/-, CD2+/-, CD5+/-, CD7-/+, CD4>CD8 may be CD4-, CD8-, may be CD45RA+ and CD45RO-.

Diagnostic problems

In marrows with interstitial involvement it may be difficult to decide whether or not the T cells are truly neoplastic. When only a marrow sample is available for diagnosis it may be impossible to reach a conclusion without parallel molecular investigations.

> **Summary of key points**
> - Histological classification of T cell lymphomas is difficult.
> - The REAL classification groups together a number of lymphomas previously recognized as separate entities in other classifications.
> - Histological grading of T cell lymphomas is less predictive of clinical behaviour than histological grading of B cell lymphomas.

Angioimmunoblastic lymphoma (AIL)

Chapter 8.15

General features

This is an uncommon condition which is clinically distinct and has a variable clinical course with occasional remissions and relapses, but often transforming into a frank high-grade lymphoma (mostly T cell but occasionally B cell). Patients usually have fever, generalized lymphadenopathy, skin rash and raised polyclonal gammaglobulins.

Histopathology of the bone marrow

The diagnosis of angioimmunoblastic lymphoma requires a lymph node biopsy (Fig. 8.102). The marrow is involved in a significant number of cases (Fig. 8.103). Focal areas of fibrosis and increased vascularization are seen though the complex arborizing vasculature with PAS-positive walls seen in affected lymph nodes is much less obvious and may be absent. Within these areas a highly polymorphic cell population is found. Reactive and neoplastic cells are intimately admixed and include plasma cells, eosinophils, epithelioid macrophages together with the neoplastic small and medium sized lymphocytes and immunoblasts.

> **Immunophenotype:** CD2+, CD3+, CD4+/-, CD5+, CD7+, CD8-.

Diagnostic problems
Angioimmunoblastic lymphoma vs. Hodgkin's disease

The fibrosis, focal nature of the disease within the marrow and the mixed inflammatory cell infiltrate including eosinophils might indicate a diagnosis of Hodgkin's disease. The distinction will best be made on the lymph node biopsy though immunostaining will be

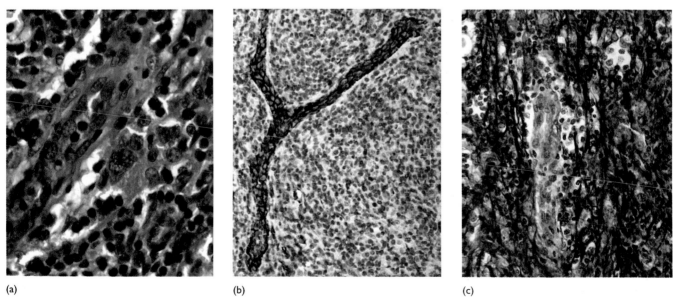

(a) (b) (c)

Fig 8.102 Lymph node involvement by AIL. (a) H&E, high power. (b) CD31 immunostain highlighting vascularity. (c) CD21 immunostain showing dendritic reticulin cell meshwork around vessels.

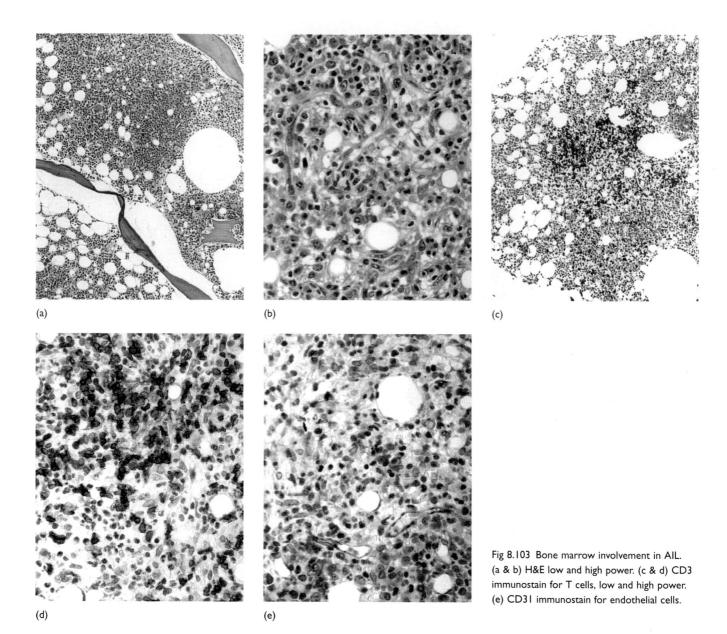

(a)

(b)

(c)

(d)

(e)

Fig 8.103 Bone marrow involvement in AIL.
(a & b) H&E low and high power. (c & d) CD3
immunostain for T cells, low and high power.
(e) CD31 immunostain for endothelial cells.

helpful if no other material is available. In AILD the abnormal large cells are usually T cells (but occasionally B cells) with little expression of CD30 and no CD15 positivity.

Angioimmunoblastic lymphoma vs. mastocytosis

Mastocytosis may also involve the marrow in a similar way and a mixed inflammatory infiltrate is not uncommon. The fibrosis and increased number of endothelial cells may produce an appearance of a spindled cell population in angioimmunoblastic lymphoma similar to the spindled mast cells in mastocytosis. The mast cell granules are likely to be identified in most instances of mastocytosis on the Giemsa stain. Immunostaining for T cell (CD3) and

macrophage (CD68; positive in mastocytosis) markers will also be helpful.

Summary of key points
- Angioimmunoblastic lymphoma has a variable clinical course.
- Marrow lesions lack the characteristic architectural features seen in lymph nodes.
- Differential diagnosis includes Hodgkin's disease and mastocytosis.

Adult T cell lymphoma/leukaemia

General features

This is a rare condition in the West and was originally described in patients from Japan and later the Caribbean. It is caused by the human T cell lymphotropic virus (HTLV 1), a type C retrovirus. It usually involves adults and has an aggressive course with leukaemia, hypercalcaemia, hepatosplenomegaly and lytic bone lesions. Rare cases with an indolent clinical course and mild lymphocytosis have been described. Patients have antibodies to HTLV 1. Characteristic clover leaf lymphocytes are seen in the peripheral blood.

Histopathology of the bone marrow

The marrow is involved in the majority of cases and tends to have a diffuse pattern which ranges from sparse to packed. There is marked cellular pleomorphism and the variation in cell size from case to case is great (Fig. 8.104).

Large cells may resemble Reed–Sternberg cells. Mitotic figures are easily found. Increased osteoclast activity with bone resorption may be seen, even in the absence of a demonstrable lymphoma infiltrate.

Reactive features include increased vascularization, eosinophils and plasma cells.

> **Immunophenotype:** CD2+, CD3+, CD4+, CD5+, CD25+, CD7-

Diagnostic problems

Serological investigation for HTLV antibodies in suspected cases will confirm or refute the diagnosis. On histological grounds alone it may not be possible to distinguish adult T cell lymphoma

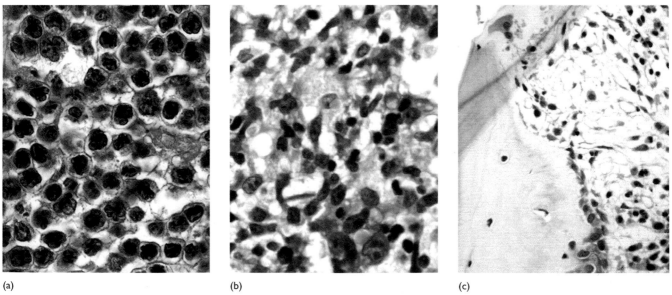

(a)   (b)   (c)

Fig 8.104. The marrow may be diffusely infiltrated by pleomorphic cells (a) or they may be scattered (b). Typically, increased osteoblastic and osteoclastic activity is present (c).

involvement of the marrow from other T cell lymphoma infiltrates. The presence of Reed–Sternberg-like cells in some cases should not lead to a misdiagnosis of Hodgkin's disease because the associated neoplastic infiltrate of small and medium-sized pleomorphic cells would not be a feature of Hodgkin's disease. In cases where there is still doubt the clinical picture of a leukaemia will readily make the distinction.

Rare cases of adult T cell lymphoma without leukaemia have been reported and this possibility should be borne in mind in cases with an atypical clinical presentation.

Summary of key points
- Adult T cell lymphoma is caused by a retrovirus, HTLV 1.
- The disease is usually clinically aggressive.
- The marrow is involved to varying degrees in the majority of patients.
- The neoplastic cells tend to be highly pleomorphic.
- Patients will have antibodies to HTLV 1.

Anaplastic large cell lymphoma Chapter 8.17

General features

This is a recently recognized entity whose identity was revealed by antibody Ki-1(CD30). In addition to expressing the activated lymphocyte antigen CD30, many cases (up to 75% in some series) are positive with T cell markers. Other cases express either B cell antigens or are non-B non-T (so-called 'null cell' cases). Most of the T cell and a proportion of the null cases have a translocation between chromosome 2 and 5 juxtaposing two genes, nucleophosmin (NPM) and anaplastic lymphoma kinase (ALK), creating a new fusion protein p80. This translocation has not been reported on B cell cases which may indicate that these are a different entity. Lacking sufficient evidence on the B cell cases, the REAL classification has placed these with the diffuse large B cell lymphomas, at least for the time being.

There appears to be two forms of the disease

1 The systemic form may involve lymph nodes or extranodal sites, e.g. soft tissue, bone and skin, and behaves in a clinically aggressive manner similar to the other large cell lymphomas. It usually arises *de novo* but a few cases have occurred in patients with pre-existing Hodgkin's disease. It has a bimodal age distribution, i.e. older children and the elderly, and may possibly have a better prognosis in children than other childhood high-grade large cell lymphomas.

2 The primary cutaneous form tends to occur in adults and has a rather indolent and incurable course although it may spontaneously regress. It may be related to lymphomatoid papulosis type A.

Although anaplastic large cell lymphoma (ALCL) has only recently been characterized as an entity, it is of course not a new disease and has probably been misdiagnosed as a number of different conditions in the past, such as metastatic carcinoma, amelanotic melanoma, lymphocyte-depleted Hodgkin's disease, malignant histiocytosis, sarcoma and regressing atypical histiocytosis.

Histopathology of the bone marrow

The neoplastic cells have a distinctive morphology. They are large, have abundant cytoplasm and large pleomorphic nuclei with prominent multiple eosinophilic nucleoli. The irregular nuclear contours have led to varied fanciful descriptions such as 'jellyfish', 'embryo' and 'foot-print' like. The cells appear to adhere to each other resulting in a cohesive growth pattern. Large sheets of cells often occur and impart a syncytial appearance. Mitotic figures are easily seen. Marrow involvement is rarely subtle and a focal or diffuse pattern is seen. The diagnosis rests on the immunohistochemistry (Fig. 8.105).

Immunophenotype: CD30+, EMA+/-, CD45-/+, CD25+/-, CD15-/+, CD3+/-, p80+/-

---

Diagnostic problems

As mentioned previously, the cohesive growth pattern of this lymphoma means that it is often mistaken morphologically for metastatic carcinoma. In addition, the positivity for EMA and negativity for leucocyte common antigen (CD45) in most cases, enlarge this diagnostic trap. A wider panel of antibodies, to include anti-cytokeratins and CD30, normally permits a distinction between these two conditions. Anti-melanoma markers, e.g. S-100 and HMB45, should also be included.

It is now recognized that there is an association between Hodgkin's disease and anaplastic large cell lymphoma. Indeed, some cases have features of both and have been provisionally categorized in the REAL classification as ALCL Hodgkin's-like (Hodgkin's-related). These lymphomas have an identical immunophenotype to ALCL and are believed to behave in a particularly aggressive fashion. Identification of this entity or separation of classical ALCL from classical Hodgkin's disease is rarely a diagnostic problem in the marrow biopsy since the nodal or extranodal tissue will usually have provided the primary diagnosis.

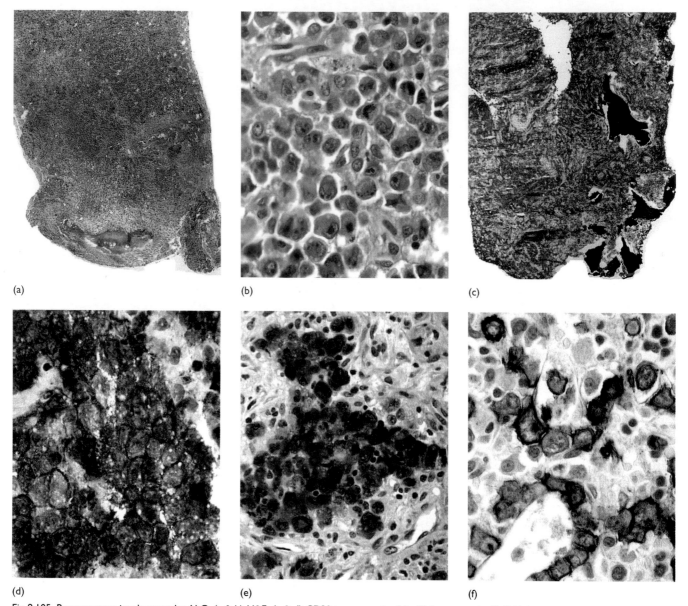

(a)

(b)

(c)

(d)

(e)

(f)

Fig 8.105 Bone marrow involvement by ALC. (a & b) H&E. (c & d) CD30 immunostain. (e) p80 immunostain. (f) EMA immunostain.

Summary of key points
- ALCL has a characteristic morphology and immunophenotype.
- ALCL has two clinical forms: systemic and primary cutaneous.
- Its cohesive growth pattern may mimic metastatic carcinoma.
- An unclear relationship between ALCL and Hodgkin's disease exists.

Hodgkin's disease

Chapter 9

Introduction

Hodgkin's disease is a lymphoma characterized by the presence of large binucleate Reed–Sternberg cells in a background of reactive-appearing lymphocytes, macrophages, granulocytes and fibroblasts. Its aetiology is unknown and the nature of the abnormal cells remains unclear though there is more evidence that they are related to B cells than any other member of the lymphoid family. The REAL classification divides Hodgkin's disease into lymphocyte predominance and classical varieties (mixed cellularity, nodular sclerosing and lymphocyte depletion).

It is now clear that lymphocyte predominance is a separate entity and is a form of B cell follicular proliferation. A question mark still remains over whether the condition is reactive or neoplastic although it undoubtedly has a predisposition to develop into a large B cell lymphoma.

The classical varieties are the same as those categorized in the 1966 RYE classification though lymphocyte depletion has become an uncommon diagnosis with most cases being reclassified as anaplastic large cell lymphomas.

Clinical

Hodgkin's disease usually presents with painless enlargement of one or more groups of lymph nodes. A history of lymph node enlargement for several weeks or months is not uncommon. The affected lymph nodes may already be quite large when first noticed, and subsequent growth may often be negligible, or the nodes may shrink or fluctuate in size. The enlarged lymph nodes are firm, non-tender, and often feel rubbery. Non-specific haematological abnormalities are common but bone marrow involvement at presentation is uncommon (especially now that so many cases previously diagnosed as lymphocyte depletion have been reclassified as non-Hodgkin lymphomas). Hodgkin's disease in the bone marrow is more frequent at relapse.

Histopathology of the bone marrow
Classical Hodgkin's disease

The bone marrow appearances of mixed cellularity or nodular sclerosis are indistinguishable so that subtyping as recommended in the original RYE classification must be performed on a lymph node biopsy. Usually the marrow shows focal involvement emphasizing the importance of an adequate-sized trephine specimen when staging Hodgkin's disease. In most cases of nodal disease with spread to the marrow, diagnostic cells are rare (Fig. 9.1) but a combination of focal fibrosis and abnormal mononuclear cells (RS cells are not essential if node involvement has been confirmed histologically) with appropriate immunostaining will allow a confident diagnosis. (Fig. 9.2) It is frequently useful to include antibodies recognizing megakaryocytes to be certain that the abnormal cells are truly derived from Hodgkin's disease.

It is very unusual for Hodgkin's disease of any subtype to present solely as a bone marrow infiltration. In such cases it will be essential to identify a definite Reed–Sternberg cell.

Lymphocyte predominance Hodgkin's disease

Since the recognition of this condition as a separate entity it is doubtful whether bone marrow involvement occurs other than when there has been a transformation to a large B cell lymphoma.

Immunophenotype:	
Classical Reed–Sternberg cells:	CD15+, CD30+,CD45-, EMA-, J chain- B cell antigens rare (except CD20)
Lymphocyte predominance (L&H) cells:	CD15-, CD30-,CD45+, EMA+/-, J chain+ B cell antigens +

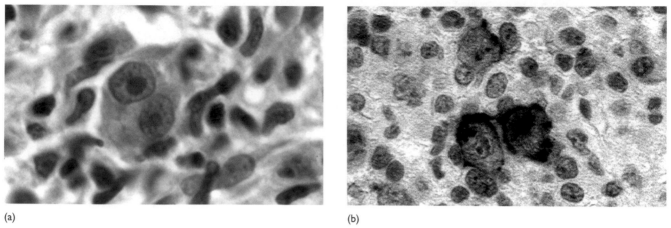

Fig 9.1 Diagnostic Reed–Sternberg cell in the bone marrow. (a) H&E. (b) Immunostain for CD30.

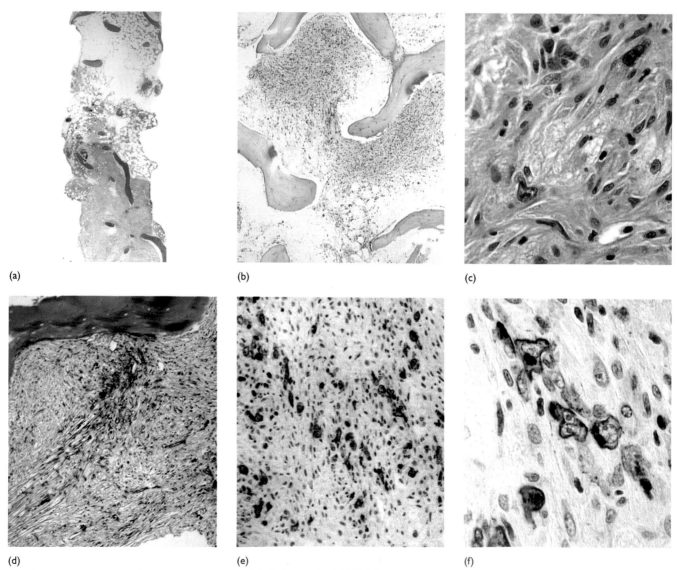

Fig 9.2 Typical involvement of the bone marrow by Hodgkin's disease. (a–c) H&E. (d) Reticulin. (e & f) Immunostain for CD30.

Diagnostic problems
Other fibrosing conditions
Superficially the abnormal cells in fibrosing myeloproliferative conditions and secondary carcinoma can look like Hodgkin cells. The key to avoiding these errors is not to diagnose Hodgkin's disease on a marrow alone without careful clinical review of the case. Appropriate immunostaining for megakaryocytes and epithelial cells should be undertaken in addition to that for Hodgkin's disease.

Summary of key points
- Classical Hodgkin's disease causes a fibrotic response typically patchy in the bone marrow.
- Involvement of the marrow is rare at presentation but relatively common at relapse.
- Immunocytochemical examination is helpful in distinguishing it from other fibrosing conditions of the bone marrow.

Metastatic disease

Chapter   10

Introduction

Metastatic spread of carcinoma and sarcoma to the bone marrow is relatively common as a terminal event when there is usually little or no clinical justification for a biopsy. In practice the number of trephines taken for diagnosis of secondary disease including those discovered by chance is small. In our own practice the last 3200 bone marrow trephines contained only 39 diagnoses of metastatic disease which is only a little over 1% of cases.

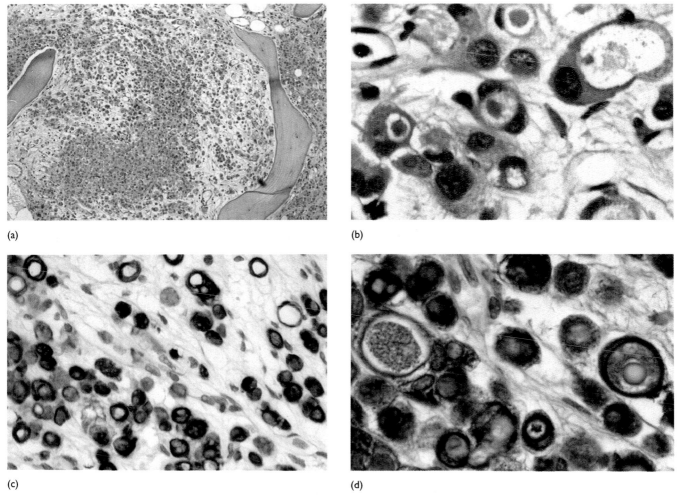

(a)

(b)

(c)

(d)

Fig 10.1 Secondary breast cancer in the bone marrow. (a & b) H&E. (c) Cytokeratin immunostain. (d) Epithelial membrane antigen (EMA) immunostain.

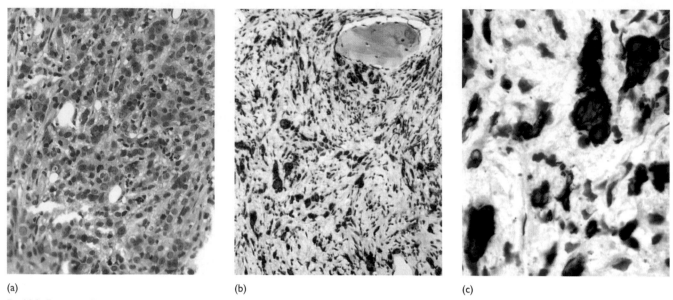

(a)   (b)   (c)

Fig 10.2 Extensive fibrosis in the marrow from secondary cancer of unknown origin. (a) H&E. (b & c) Cytokeratin immunostain.

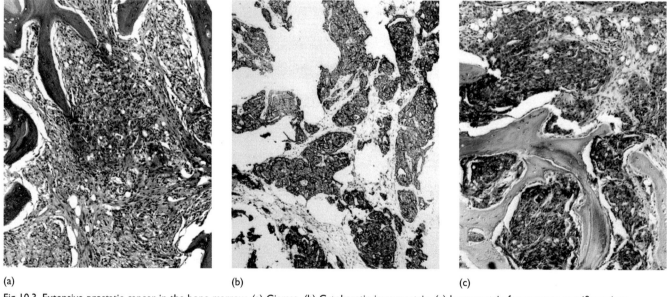

(a)   (b)   (c)

Fig 10.3 Extensive prostatic cancer in the bone marrow. (a) Giemsa. (b) Cytokeratin immunostain. (c) Immunostain for prostate specific antigen.

Clinical

Except in paediatric diseases staging biopsies are rarely taken in the UK. Most biopsies are for unexplained anaemias or localized bone pain when a diagnosis of myeloma is part of the differential. Often a leucoerythroblastic blood picture (characterized by circulating immature granulocytes, nucleated red cells, abnormal platelets and teardrop erythrocytes) is also present.

Histopathology of the bone marrow
Carcinoma

The bone marrow is virtually always grossly abnormal even at low power. Either the marrow will be heavily infiltrated by recognizable tumour (Fig. 10.1) or extensively fibrosed (Fig. 10.2). In both cases immunocytochemistry is useful to ensure that lymphoma is not overlooked. Occasionally the site of the primary tumour is unclear

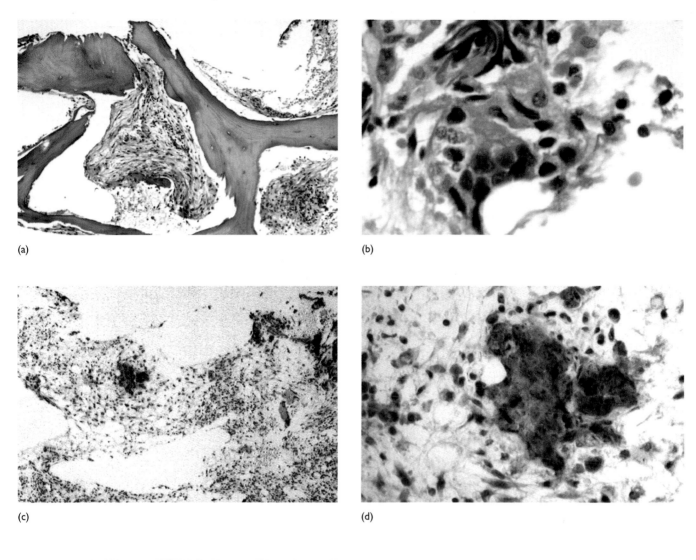

(a)

(b)

(c)

(d)

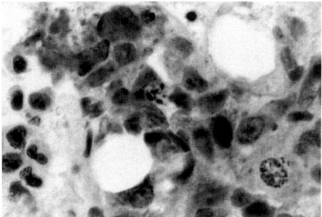

(e)

Fig 10.4 Focal involvement of bone marrow by prostatic cancer. (a & b) H&E, note bony sclerosis. (c & d) Immunostain for cytokeratin. (e) Immunostain for prostate specific antigen.

clinically so that immunostaining for endocrine and prostatic antigens can be helpful (Figs 10.3 and 10.4).

Several studies have shown that multiple biopsies taken at first presentation with a tumour such as breast cancer will demonstrate micrometastases in a proportion of cases. The relevance of these findings to clinical practice or prognosis remains unclear.

Paediatric tumours

Bone marrow trephines are taken as part of most oncology protocols for the assessment of solid tumours in childhood. Children with disseminated disease are usually identified by the clinician so marrow involvement is rarely a surprise. The differential diagnosis mainly involves neuroblastoma (and its variants), rhabdomyosarcoma and Ewing's tumour. It is very uncommon to find such tumours unexpectedly but if this arises a small panel of antibodies aimed at the 'small round blue cell tumours of childhood' will usually solve any problems (Figs 10.5 and 10.6).

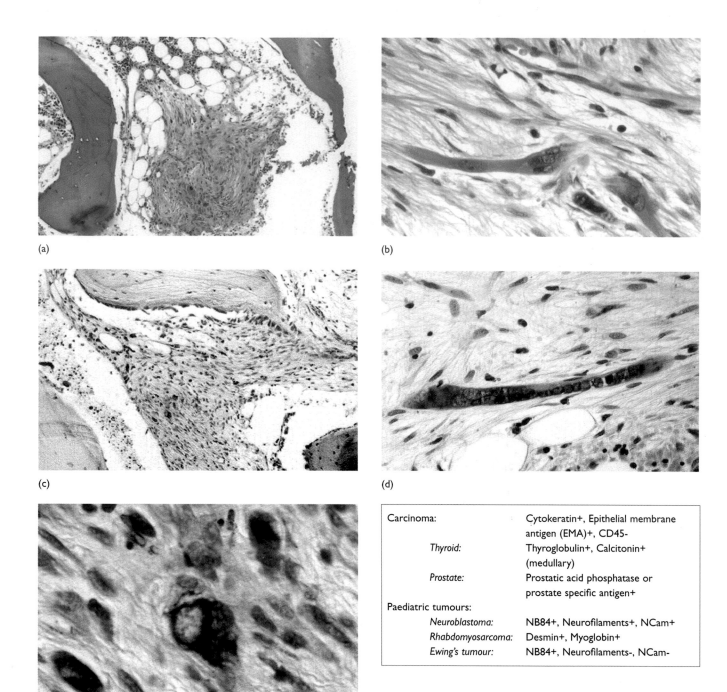

(a)

(b)

(c)

(d)

(e)

Fig 10.5 Involvement of the bone marrow by rhabdomyosarcoma.
(a & b) H&E. (c–e) Immunostain for desmin.

Carcinoma:		Cytokeratin+, Epithelial membrane antigen (EMA)+, CD45-
	Thyroid:	Thyroglobulin+, Calcitonin+ (medullary)
	Prostate:	Prostatic acid phosphatase or prostate specific antigen+
Paediatric tumours:		
	Neuroblastoma:	NB84+, Neurofilaments+, NCam+
	Rhabdomyosarcoma:	Desmin+, Myoglobin+
	Ewing's tumour:	NB84+, Neurofilaments-, NCam-

Diagnostic problems
Other fibrosing conditions

It is important not to diagnose any fibrotic marrow in a patient with a known history of carcinoma as having metastatic disease without supporting proof such as clear-cut tumour in the marrow or immunocytochemical identification of infiltrating cells. Patients with carcinoma can and do get other diseases such as myelofibrosis.

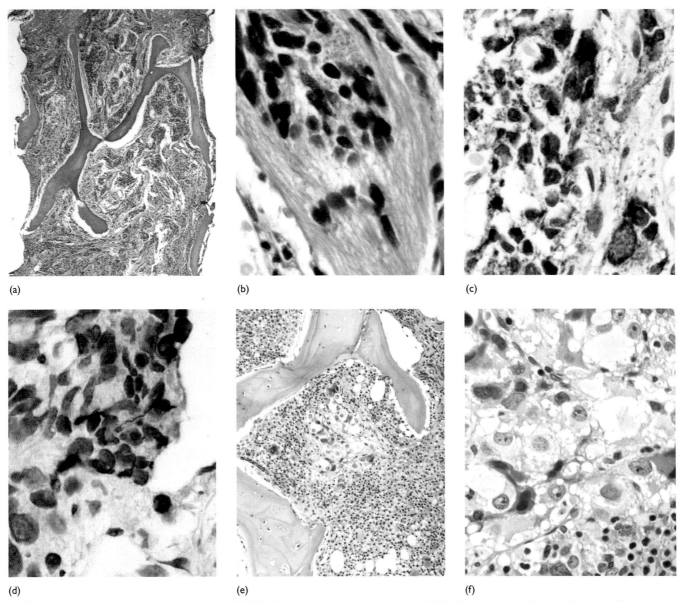

Fig 10.6 Neuroblastoma in the bone marrow. (a & b) H&E. (c) Immunostain for neural marker NB84. (d) Immunostain for neurofilaments. Occasionally neuroblastoma may be present in a differentiated form as ganglioneuroblastoma. (e & f) H&E.

Summary of key points
- Metastatic disease is a relatively uncommon indication for a bone marrow trephine.
- Involvement of the marrow is usually obvious.
- Immunocytochemical examination is helpful in distinguishing it from other fibrosing conditions of the bone marrow and in identifying different types of tumour.

Miscellaneous

Chapter   11

This chapter brings together those conditions which do not warrant chapters of their own.

Amyloidosis

This is a rare finding in a marrow biopsy. The amount of amyloid present is variable and the histological changes may be subtle requiring a high index of suspicion for its detection. It is present in the walls of vessels and also within the stroma surrounding the haematopoietic tissue. As in other tissues it is extracellular and can be demonstrated histochemically using the Congo-Red stain. This stains the amyloid orange and displays a brilliant light green colour under polarized light (Fig. 11.1). In marrows containing amyloid derived from immunoglobulin light chain, a neoplastic clone of plasma cells may also be detected.

Immune thrombocytopaenic purpura (ITP)

ITP is due to the removal of antibody-coated platelets from the circulation. The auto-antibodies are produced by the body in a number of different circumstances, the most common being:

(a) autoimmune disorders, e.g. SLE (systemic lupus erythematosus);

(b) viral infections, e.g. HIV, EBV, CMV;

(c) drug induced, e.g. carbamazepine, chlorothiazide;

(d) lymphoproliferative disorders, e.g. Hodgkin's disease, CLL;

(e) idiopathic, i.e. of unknown origin.

The acute presentation of ITP is usually seen in children as a dramatic though transitory disease usually associated with a preceding viral illness. The bone marrow is rarely biopsied. The chronic form of ITP occurs in adults and is often biopsied to eliminate dysplasias and malignancies. The marrow is relatively normal apart from an increased number of megakaryocytes which occasionally can be quite dramatic. The megakaryocytes tend to be smaller than normal and are less mature with fewer lobes than mature forms, reflecting the reactive nature of this condition (Fig. 11.2).

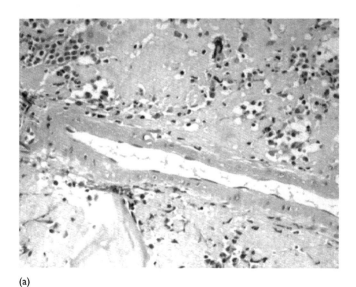
(a)

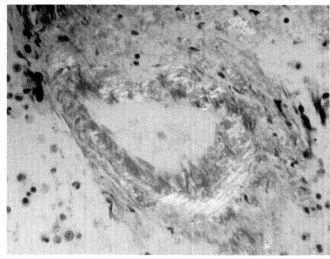
(b)

Fig 11.1 Amyloidosis in bone marrow. (a) H&E. (b) Congo Red under polarized light.

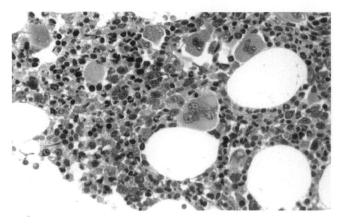

Fig 11.2 Increased numbers of small megakaryocytes in chronic ITP. Giemsa.

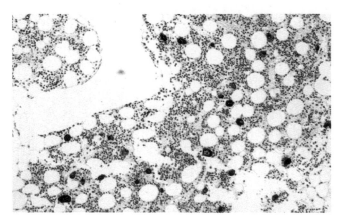

Fig 11.3 Increased numbers of megakaryocytes in ITP are easier to detect by immunostaining (CD31 in this case).

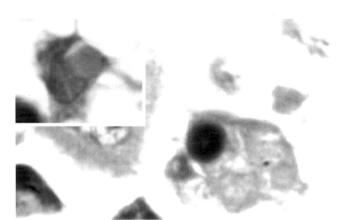

Fig 11.4 Erythrophagocytosis: macrophage stuffed with erythrocytes compared with an example containing a single red cell (insert). Giemsa.

Table 11.1 Pathological conditions often associated with erythrophagocytosis.

Viral infections, e.g. infectious mononucleosis
Bacterial infections
Haemolytic anaemia
AIDS
Familial erythrophagocytic lymphohistiocytosis
Malignancy, e.g. T cell lymphoma
Post-chemotherapy
Malignant histiocytosis (very rare and erythrophagocytosis is not prominent)

Table 11.2 Causes of fibrosis in the bone marrow.

Common	Less common
Myeloproliferative disease	Acute leukaemias
• Chronic primary myelofibrosis	Treated acute leukaemias
• Acute myelofibrosis (acute megakaryoblastic leukaemia)	Systemic mastocytosis
• Polycythaemia rubra vera	Myelodysplasia
• Essential thrombocythaemia	Non-Hodgkin's lymphoma, e.g.
• Chronic granulocytic leukaemia	• Multiple myeloma
Hodgkin's disease	• Waldenström's macroglobulinaemia
Metastatic carcinoma	Tuberculosis
	Sarcoidosis
	Scarring; following necrosis, previous biopsy, fracture, osteomyelitis
	Paget's disease
	Renal osteodystrophy

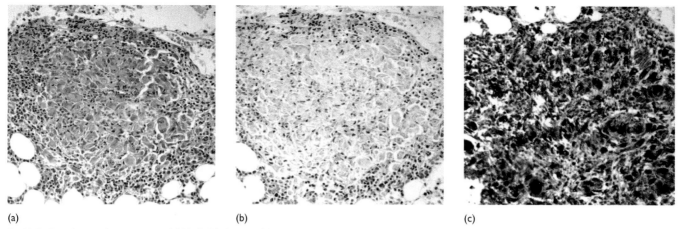

(a)   (b)   (c)

Fig 11.5 Granuloma in bone marrow. (a) H&E. (b) Giemsa. (c) Immunostain for CD68 (macrophage marker).

Table 11.3 Causes of granulomas.

Infection	• Histoplasmosis	**Sarcoidosis**	• Ibuprofen
• Tuberculosis	• Cryptococcosis	**Malignant disease**	• Indomethacin
• Atypical mycobacteria	• Saccharomyces	• Hodgkin's disease	• Allopurinol
• Disseminated BCG	• Blastomycosis	• Multiple myeloma	• Interferon alpha-2b
• Brucellosis	• Coccidioidomycosis	• Non-Hodgkin's lymphoma	
• Leprosy	• Paracoccidioidomycosis	• Mycosis fungoides	**Post-transplantation of bone**
• Syphilis	• Infectious mononucleosis	• ALL	**marrow**
• Typhoid fever	• CMV	• MDS	**Associated with eosinophilic**
• Legionnaire's disease	• Herpes zoster	**Drug hypersensitivity**	**interstitial nephritis**
• Tularaemia	• Hantaan virus	• Phenytoin	**Renal osteodystrophy**
• Q fever	• Cat scratch fever	• Procainamide	**Reaction to foreign**
• Rocky Mountain Spotted	• Viral hepatitis	• Phenylbutazone &	**substances**
fever		oxyphenylbutazone	• Anthracosis and silicosis
• Leishmaniasis		• Chlorpropamide	• Talc
• Toxoplasmosis		• Sulphasalazine	• Berylliosis

It is generally easy to distinguish ITP from myelodysplasia and myeloproliferation by its lack of architectural and cytological abnormality.

Assessing the number of megakaryocytes in a marrow trephine can be done by formal counting and normal ranges are quoted (12–25 megakaryocytes per sq. mm[1,2]). In practice a significant increase (i.e. more than twice the normal upper range) in megakaryocyte numbers can be confidently identified with a little experience of trephine histology or by immunostaining (Fig. 11.3).

Erythrophagocytosis

Occasional examples of red cells phagocytosed by macrophages can be found in most marrows if one is prepared to spend the time looking. Erythrophagocytosis refers to those conditions (Table 11.1) where many if not the majority of the macrophages contain phagocytosed red cells, sometimes being stuffed with them (Fig. 11.4).

Fibrosis

The causes of fibrosis in the bone marrow are numerous (Table 11.2). A semiquantitative method of assessment is described in Chapter 2 (p. 7).

Granulomas

As with other tissues in the body, granulomas in the marrow can have a wide variety of appearances, ranging from occasional collections of a few epithelioid macrophages to fully formed granulomas consisting of tight clusters of epithelioid macrophages and multinucleated giant cells with a cuff of small lymphocytes. It is our experience that granulomas are easier to identify using H&E rather than Giemsa which tends to stain epithelioid macrophages poorly (Fig. 11.5). There are numerous causes (Table 11.3) for granuloma formation and the pathologist can often only provide a differential diagnosis relevant to the clinical details. In a percentage of cases no cause will ever be found.

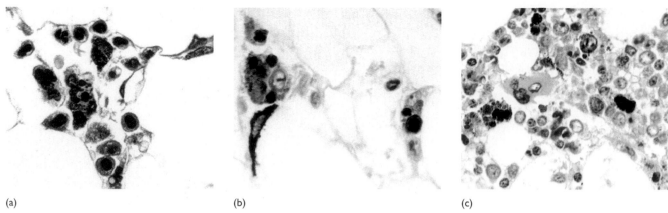

(a)　　　　　　　　　　　　　　(b)　　　　　　　　　　　　　　(c)

Fig 11.6 Iron in macrophages following blood transfusion. (a) H&E. (b & c) Giemsa.

Table 11.4 Semiquantitative grading scheme for haemosiderin in tissue section. After Krause et al.[3]

Grade	Appearance
0	No iron seen
1	Granules in 1 out of 3 high powered fields
2	Granules in 1 out of 2 high powered fields
3	A few granules in every high powered field
4	> a few granules in every high powered field

Table 11.5 Conditions affecting iron stores.

Lack of iron due to:
- chronic disease
- inadequate diet
- chronic bleeding
- polycythaemia vera

Excess iron due to:
- aplasia
- leukaemia
- multiple transfusions, e.g. thalassaemia
- MDS
- chronic disease with impaired iron handling and accumulation in macrophages

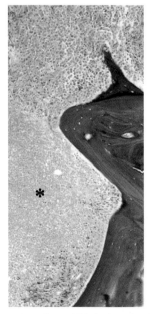

Fig 11.7 Necrosis: transition from viable leukaemia cells to total necrosis (*). Giemsa.

Haemosiderin

Haemosiderin can be detected in both H&E and Giemsa stained sections. It takes the form of fine and coarse granules which appear brown on H&E and olive green on Giemsa stained sections (Fig. 11.6).

The granules are present within macrophages and may be associated with erythroid colonies. Decalcification of the biopsy may reduce the amount of iron so that assessment of iron content is best done on the aspirate smear. A semiquantitative method of assessing iron content is shown in Table 11.4.

The most commonly encountered conditions which may affect iron stores are listed in Table 11.5.

Necrosis

When examining a marrow trephine, it is important to make the distinction between

1 necrosis involving the bone and marrow, such as is seen in sickle cell disease, embolism, caisson disease (the 'bends'), sepsis, and

2 necrosis predominantly affecting the marrow tissue, which is almost invariably associated with malignancy, such as acute

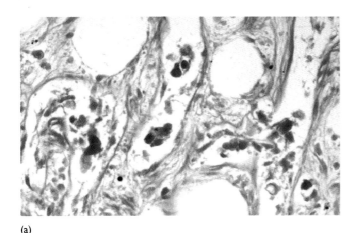

(a)

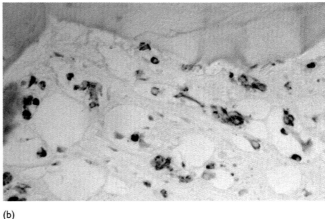

(b)

Fig 11.8 Necrotic carcinoma cells in bone marrow can be clearly identified by immunostaining for cytokeratins. (a) H&E. (b) Immunostain for cytokeratins.

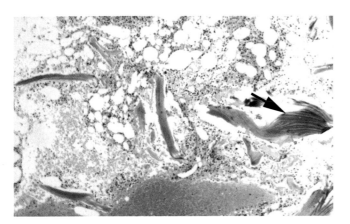

Fig 11.9 Osteoporosis: typical thin easily fractured trabeculae. Note the osteoid seams are relatively normal (arrow). Giemsa.

leukaemia, non Hodgkin's lymphoma, Hodgkin's disease and metastatic carcinoma. If the tumour load in the marrow is high and there is massive necrosis then the bone may also become involved. Dead bone is identified by loss of the osteocyte population.

The necrotic cells show the features of necrosis seen in any tissue. The cells initially have darkly staining pyknotic nuclei which later disintegrate as karyorrhexis and karyolysis occurs. The cytoplasm is smudgy and eosinophilic. The overall impression is of ghost-like cells lacking any sharp well-defined features. Areas of fibrosis may be seen as healing occurs (Fig. 11.7).

Immunohistochemistry may be useful in identifying the nature of the dead cells, e.g. anti-cytokeratin antibodies have been shown to be useful in this respect. Care must be taken in interpretation of immunohistochemistry because of the increased tendency for antibodies to adhere in a nonspecific way to necrotic tissue (Fig. 11.8).

Osteoporosis

Osteoporosis is a decreased amount of bone per unit volume. This results in a reduction in the amount of trabecular bone seen in a tissue section by a thinning of the trabeculae. Morphometry of bone will allow an accurate assessment of bone trabecular thickness but as a general rule a trabecula is at least the width of a fat cell. However, trabecular thickness varies individually and unless the condition is severe it is not that easy to identify osteoporosis in a routine trephine. A useful guide comes from a trephine where the bones are fragmented (because they are so weak) but the rest of the marrow is well preserved (indicating good technical preservation). Usually in these cases the clinician has already identified the condition by its feel at biopsy (Fig. 11.9).

Osteoporotic change is most frequently seen in the elderly population especially in women. It is also seen in bones no longer stimulated by normal weight-bearing activities, e.g. patients who are immobilized.

Less common causes include endocrine disorders, long-term steroid administration and certain malignancies, e.g. multiple myeloma.

Renal osteodystrophy

Renal osteodystrophy or renal bone disease is caused by the metabolic changes associated with chronic renal failure such as hypocalcaemia and secondary hyperparathyroidism. This is a complex bony abnormality which may include the changes of osteomalacia, osteitis fibrosa cystica, osteoporosis and osteosclerosis either singly or in combinations.

Bone marrow biopsies from patients with chronic renal failure may show a number of histological changes related to this constellation of conditions. There is usually evidence of increased destruction of bone and increased production. These structural changes are seen in association with abnormal cellular activity in the form of

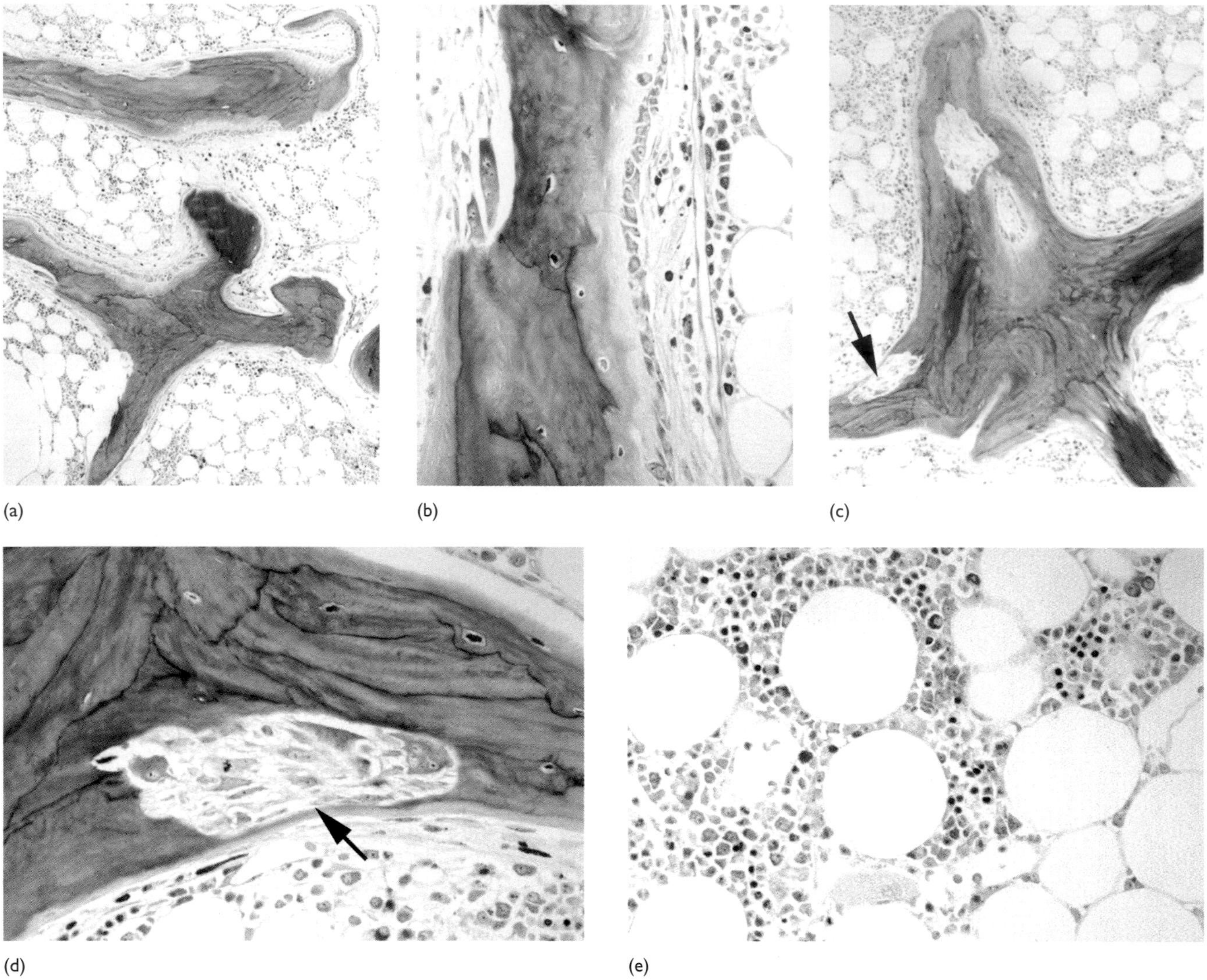

Fig 11.10 Typical renal bone disease; see text for details of changes. (a – d) illustrate the constellation of changes in the bones with examples of tunnelling (arrows) in c, d. (e) is a higher power of the marrow showing mild erythroid hyperplasia. Giemsa.

increased osteoblasts and osteoclasts. The bone trabeculae may have 'tunnels' excavated within them by osteoclasts. These are essentially exaggerated forms of Howship's lacunae. These newly created spaces, and eventually the intertrabecular spaces containing the marrow, may be filled with vascularized fibrous tissue. The osteoblasts lay down new bone which is of the woven variety and there is an increase in the amount of osteoid (not apparent in decalcified sections). In extreme cases the appearances of osteodystrophy may resemble Paget's disease of the bone, although in the latter case the trabeculae are generally thicker and a mosaic pattern of cement lines is evident.

The marrow itself is unremarkable or shows erythroid hyperplasia and there may be increased haemosiderin from multiple blood transfusions for anaemia (Fig. 11.10).

Paget's disease

Paget's disease is of unknown aetiology and affects 3–4% of the population over the age of 45 years. Probably less than 5% of cases are symptomatic and may present as bone pain due to microfractures, deafness because of mechanical damage to the auditory nerve or rarely as cardiac failure. There is also an increased risk of developing osteogenic sarcoma.

The histological features are:

1 Increased osteoclastic activity in the early stages with marked resorption of bone as evidenced by numerous Howship's lacunae containing large multinucleated osteoclasts.

2 This is followed by bone hyperplasia undertaken by increased numbers of osteoblasts. The bone is laid down, originally as woven bone and then as lamellar bone. This results in thickened trabecu-

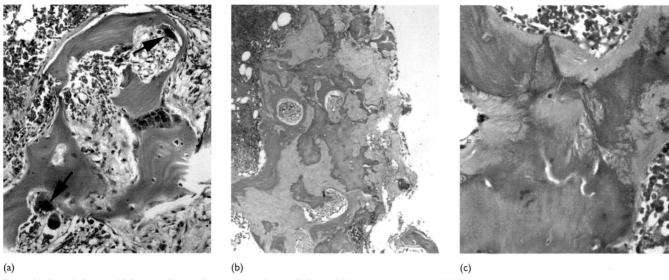

(a)   (b)   (c)

Fig 11.11 Paget's disease. (a) Increased osteoclastic activity (arrows). (b & c) Mosaic bone pattern. All H&E.

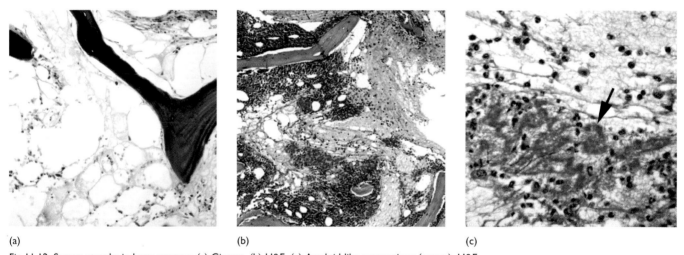

(a)   (b)   (c)

Fig 11.12 Serous atrophy in bone marrow. (a) Giemsa. (b) H&E. (c) Amyloid-like aggregations (arrow), H&E.

lae with disjointed, multidirectional cement lines: the so-called mosaic pattern.

3 Within the marrow space there is an increase in the vascularity, which if extensive can act as an arterio-venous shunt resulting occasionally in high output cardiac failure (Fig. 11.11).

Serous atrophy

This has also been termed gelatinous transformation and serous degeneration. It was originally described in patients with anorexia nervosa but may be seen in anyone with rapid marked loss in body weight (Table 11.6). Nowadays it is frequently seen in patients with AIDS who have had severe weight loss. The changes are usually focal with the marrow fat cells being surrounded and gradually replaced by an extracellular homogeneous fibrillary pale material which is rich in hyaluronic acid. On H&E stained sections it has a smoky lilac colour, sometimes with brighter red aggregations which should be distinguished from amyloid (Fig. 11.12).

Vasculitis

The marrow has a rich blood supply and contains a range of blood vessel types, including small arteries, which are susceptible to the same diseases that affect blood vessels elsewhere in the body. It is not particularly well endowed with the medium to large vessels which are more commonly affected by the major forms of vasculi-

Table 11.6 Causes of serous atrophy (gelatinous transformation of the marrow).

AIDS	Anorexia nervosa
Cancer	Chemotherapy
Chronic renal disease	Hypothroidism
Irradiation	Malabsorption
TB	

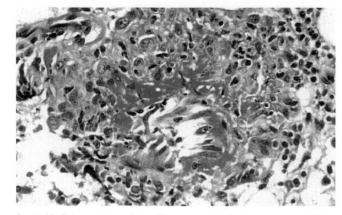

Fig 11.13 Polyarteritis nodosa affecting arteriole in bone marrow. H&E.

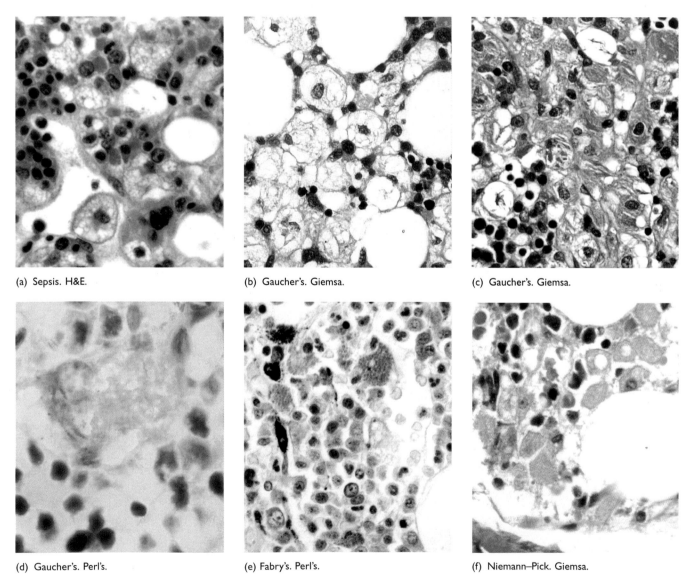

(a) Sepsis. H&E.

(b) Gaucher's. Giemsa.

(c) Gaucher's. Giemsa.

(d) Gaucher's. Perl's.

(e) Fabry's. Perl's.

(f) Niemann–Pick. Giemsa.

Fig 11.14 Foamy macrophages in various conditions.

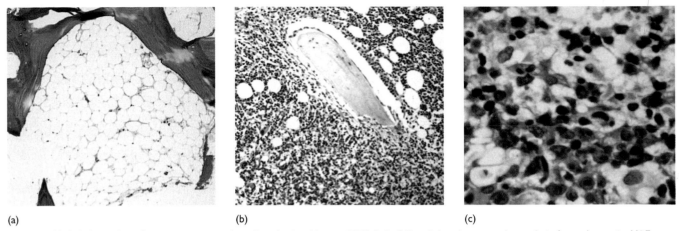

(a)   (b)   (c)

Fig 11.15 (a) Aplasia resulting from exposure to solvent-based paint thinners, H&E. (b & c) Pseudolymphomatous hyperplasia from phenytoin, H&E.

Table 11.7 Conditions in which foamy macrophages may be seen.

Sepsis, e.g. occasionally seen in ITU patients
Fat necrosis, e.g. may be related to previous biopsy at that site
Hyperlipidaemia
Pseudo-Gaucher cells
Inherited disorders
• Gaucher's disease
• Niemann–Pick disease
• Fabry's disease
• Batten's disease
Histiocytosis X

tis so the trephine rarely yields a positive diagnosis. Occasionally it can be helpful or even diagnostic in conditions such as poly-arteritis nodosa (Fig. 11.13).

Foamy macrophages

Foamy macrophages are seen in a number of very different conditions (Table 11.7). In severe sepsis the macrophages contain lipid vacuoles, presumably derived from erythrocyte membrane degradation. Haemosiderin may also be present (Fig. 11.14).

Inherited lipid storage disorders are characterized by the presence of foamy macrophages sometimes filling the marrow as in Gaucher's disease or scattered focally as in Niemann–Pick or Fabry's disease. In certain haematological malignancies, particularly chronic myeloid leukaemia, cells resembling Gaucher's cells ('pseudo-Gaucher cells') have been described although in our experience they are not a prominent or common feature.

The effects of drugs and chemicals

Drugs and chemicals have a variety of effects on the marrow which are beyond the scope of this text (and these authors!). In many cases the changes are nonspecific, e.g. excessive intake of alcohol may produce an increase in the numbers of plasma cells and mast cells within the marrow. Others are more dramatic such as the striking aplasia that can be induced by solvent exposure or the pseudo-lymphomatous changes of phenytoin. Perhaps the most important point to make is to consider the drug history with any marrow changes inexplicable on other grounds (Fig. 11.15).

References

1 Ellis JT, Peterson P. The bone marrow in polycythemia vera. In Sommers JC (ed); *Pathology Annual* Vol. 14. Part 1. New York, Appleton-Century-Crofts, 1979, pp. 383–403.

2 Branehög I, Kutti J, Ridell B, Swolin B, Weinfeld A. The relation of thrombokinetics to bone marrow megakaryocytes in idiopathic thrombocytopenic purpura. *Blood* 1975; **45**: 551–562.

3 Krause JR, Brubaker DO, Kaplan J. Comparison of stainable iron in aspirated and needle biopsy specimens of bone marrow. *Am J Clin Pathol* 1979; **72**: 68–70.

Technical considerations

Introduction

The debate over whether trephines should be embedded in paraffin wax or plastic resin will doubtless continue for some time. We have reviewed this in some detail in Chapter 1 and given our reasons for believing that paraffin-embedding is more satisfactory for routine diagnosis. The following technical considerations mainly relate to marrow biopsies which have been embedded in paraffin wax.

Preparation of bone marrow biopsies

Whatever methods are used in preparing marrow biopsies, it is essential that:

- there be effective fixation of the tissue to ensure that good morphology is retained and that the bone is processed to enable sections of 2–4 µm to be cut;
- a range of special staining techniques (e.g. Giemsa, Reticulin) remain applicable;
- tissue antigenicity is not adversely affected by procedures so that immunohistochemical techniques are applicable.

Both the bone marrow trephine biopsy and bone marrow aspirate, i.e. clot specimen, may be used to examine the state of the marrow.

Fixation

FIXATIVE

All specimens are fixed in 2% formol-acetic, i.e.

Formaldehyde, 40% w/v	1 litre
Water	9 litres
Sodium chloride	87 g
Glacial acetic acid	200 mL

DURATION OF FIXATION

Aspirates: fixation of aspirate specimens is complete after 24 hours. The particles are embedded in 1–2% agar and processed as tissue blocks.

Trephines: Trephine specimens should be fixed for 48–72 hours and over this period the solution changed at least three times: more frequently if the trephine is large or there is a lot of bone. This is satisfactory for the majority of specimens.

Occasionally trephines are received containing a relatively large amount of solid bone or cartilage which proves an obstacle to satisfactory sectioning. In such cases that part of the core can be separated from the remainder of the tissue since it is unlikely to contain cells of diagnostic significance.

If the core contains spicules of bone that remain heavily calcified, surface decalcification (with Perenyi's fluid) after embedding may ease the situation although this must be done judiciously to prevent damage to tissue morphology or antigenicity.

Processing and embedding

Specimens are processed to paraffin wax on an automated processor using an overnight schedule (15–18 hours). They are then blocked out in paraffin wax before sectioning on a conventional microtome (Rotary, Sledge, Base sledge) at 2–4 µm using disposable blades (Feather).

Staining of bone marrow biopsies

A standard haematoxylin and eosin stain is usually satisfactory. For Giemsa staining the authors use the following recipe. As in cookery, good results require fine ingredients but will reward skill and patience.

Giemsa stain

1 Dewax and rehydrate sections (2–4 µm).
2 Wash in distilled water.
3 Place slides in Giemsa working solution for 1 hour. Stock solution: Giemsa's stain, BDH/Gurr product 35014. Working solution: dilute stock solution 1:4 with distilled water.
4 Wash well in water.
5 Commence differentiation by agitation in freshly prepared acetic acid solution, i.e. 100 mL distilled water to which 6–8 drops of glacial acetic acid has been added. Section will appear deep pink when this phase is complete.

6 Transfer directly to 95% IMS (industrial methylated spirit) and with gentle agitation, complete differentiation.

7 Halt differentiation by rinsing in iso-propyl alcohol.

8 Clear in xylene.

9 Mount in DPX (mounting medium — BDH).

Immunohistochemistry

PRETREATMENT

Microwaving

Tissue antigenicity can be enhanced by enzyme digestion and microwave heating or pressure cooking. It is therefore advisable to cut sections onto slides coated with an adhesive such as silane.

A suggested methodology for microwave retrieval of antigens which are not normally detectable in standard processed material is given below:

1 Dewax and rehydrate sections. If a technique incorporating a peroxidase label is used, block endogenous enzyme activity as usual.

2 Wash in distilled water.

3 Place slides in glass rack in a pyrex dish and immerse in sufficient solution to cover slides:

0.01 M   sodium citrate, $Na_3C_6H_5O_72H_2O$ (2.94 g/L)

0.01 M   sodium bicarbonate, $NaHCO_3$ (0.84 g/L)

0.01 M   HCl/sodium citrate buffer, pH 6.0

33 mL 0.01 M sodium citrate

+ 17 mL 0.01 M HCl

Cover dish with microwave-proof cling film. Puncture to allow steam to escape.

4 Microwave for 5 minutes at full power. Check fluid level; top up as necessary. Microwave for a further 5 minutes at full power. Remove from oven and allow slides to stand for 10–15 minutes in the hot solution.

5 Wash in distilled water and then in buffer. Proceed with immunocytochemical technique.

Disadvantages and limitations

• Sections are easily detached during the microwaving procedure. Slides coated with silane or poly-L-lysine must be used.

• Denaturation of tissue may occur, resulting in unrecognizable morphology, if exposed for excessive periods or if tissue is fixed in solutions other than formalin.

• With some antibodies, the treatment leads to staining distributions greater than that seen by other techniques, suggesting this may be artefactual.

• The method is not suitable for use with all antibodies.

It appears that heating rather than the action of microwaves is the important feature, although heating in distilled water has little effect. Heating in a pressure cooker or an autoclave gives similar results.

Pressure treatment (using a standard domestic pressure cooker)

1 Dissolve 5.88 g of sodium citrate in 2 litres of distilled water and correct pH to 6.0.

2 Pour the citrate buffer into the pressure cooker.

3 Place the lid loosely on the body of the pan and heat to a 'rolling boil'.

4 When a 'rolling boil' occurs, place the slides into the boiling buffer.*

Four racks can be used at once in most pressure cookers.

5 Seal the pan and ensure that the cook control is in the manual position.

6 The emergency pressure seal will soon rise, but it is necessary to wait another 5–8 minutes until the metal part of the Rise 'N' Time indicator has risen (a clear indicator that the correct temperature has been reached.)

7 Fill sink with cold water.

8 Once the Rise 'N' Time indicator has risen, time for 90 seconds.

9 Reduce pressure by immediately placing pan in sink and flushing the lid with cold tap water.

10 Once hissing stops and the emergency seal falls back, lid can be opened; fill pan to the brim with cold water before removing slide racks.

N.B. Boiling fluid at pressure can lead to severe burns if mishandled. — if in difficulties, leave pan on hotplate, turn off heat and do not return to pan until pressure has subsided.

The value of immunostaining methods

Alkaline phosphatase methods are particularly suited to bone marrow specimens due to their high amount of endogenous peroxidase activity. With careful suppression, equally high quality results are readily obtainable with immunoperoxidase methods. Most immunostaining procedures can be adapted to trephines and laboratories should refer to their antibody suppliers for advice and technical support.

Remember that relatively few antibodies are absolutely specific for individual cell types. It is important for pathologists to consult the specification sheet enclosed with these products or original papers before using new antibodies and it is always a good idea to perform stainings with a panel of antibodies to ensure that exceptions to general rules are observed. For example, a small number of malignant melanomas and anaplastic large cell lymphomas express cytokeratins. If appropriate confirmatory stains are not included, an incorrect diagnosis of carcinoma may be made. Below we have attempted to cover those areas of diagnostic pathology where immunohistochemistry may be most usefully applied. These are:

1 assessment of cellularity;

2 dry tap;

3 focal disease;

---

* Slides should be spaced out in the rack.

Table 12.1 Suggested antibody types for identifying normal cells.

Normal cell types	Antibody
Megakaryocytes and precursors	CD61, CD31, factor VIII-related antigen
Erythroid cells	Glycophorin A or C
Granulocytes	Neutrophil elastase, myeloperoxidase or CD15
Monocytes	CD68
Plasma cells	P63 plasma cell antigen, kappa & lambda light chains
Lymphocytes	Leucocyte common antigen CD45
Vessels	CD31, CD34 or factor VIII-related antigen

Table 12.2 Causes and diagnoses of dry taps.

Cause of dry tap	Diagnosis	Antibody types
(a) Fibrosis	Secondary carcinoma	Cytokeratin, epithelial membrane antigen
	Neuroblastoma	Neuroblastoma-associated antigen (NB84)
	Rhabdomyosarcoma	Desmin or myoglobin
	Hodgkin's disease	CD15 or CD30
(b) Hypercellular	Lymphoma	See section 4 *Classification of lymphoma and leukaemia*
	Leukaemia	See section 4 *Classification of lymphoma and leukaemia*
	Reactive*	CD61 → megakaryocytes
		Elastase → granulocytes
		Glycophorin A or C → erythroid
		p63 antigen → plasma cells

* The reason for utilizing these antibodies is to eliminate the malignant causes of hypercellularity by showing that the cells present are normal marrow components.

4 classification of lymphoma and leukaemia.

1 *Assessment of cellularity.* It is often useful to give clinicians accurate information on the cellular make-up of particular marrow samples — for example, the ratio of residual marrow cells to malignant infiltrate and the assessment of a bone marrow prior to harvest for autologous transplantation. There are a number of antibodies which are very useful in labelling individual cell lines of the haematopoietic tissue (Table 12.1).

2 *Dry tap.* A dry tap means that on aspiration of the bone, no marrow cells are obtained so that a trephine needs to be taken if diagnostic material is required. Dry tap is generally explained by a fibrotic reaction in the marrow or an increase in cellularity sufficient to prevent aspiration, i.e. a 'packed' marrow. Table 12.2 outlines the main causes of these and lists easily available antibody types which will assist in diagnosis.

3 *Focal disease.* Foci of malignant disease often cause diagnostic problems either because they are not aspirated or not spread out into the smear. Some causes of focal disease in bone marrows are shown in Table 12.3. One special problem in this area is to distinguish reactive from malignant lymphoid nodules. There is no easy solution to this problem especially if the nodules are small and composed mainly of well-differentiated small lymphocytes. Here the

only test of value is to demonstrate light chain clonality which cannot always be performed reliably regardless of the expertise of the individual laboratory.

4 *Classification of lymphoma and leukaemia.* Lymphoma classification is a complex area and differs depending on the exact scheme used by different pathologists. Table 12.4 is an outline of the results that can be achieved by immunostaining which will be of assistance in establishing the general categories of lymphomas that are recognized by most lymphoma diagnosticians. For example, most schemes now accept that lymphomas should be divided into T or B cell types. For further details consult Chapter 8.

Antibodies for diagnostic use and the CD system
Throughout this text we have referred to antigens where possible by using their CD designation. CD stands for 'Cluster of Differenti-

Table 12.3 Some causes of focal disease in bone marrows.

Lymphoma, especially follicular and CLL— see Table 12.4
Hodgkin's disease — see Table 12.2
Carcinoma — see Table 12.2

Table 12.4 Immunocytochemical aids in lymphoma and leukaemia diagnosis.

Lymphoma	Antibody types
Lymphoid origin	Leucocyte common antigen positive (except many anaplastic large cell lymphomas which are negative)
High or low grade	Proliferating cell nuclear antigen (PCNA)
	Ki-67 antigen (monoclonal and polyclonal)
B cells	CD20 or CD79a
T cells	CD3 (polyclonal) or CD45RO
Anaplastic large cell lymphoma (ALC)	CD30 and EMA
Myeloma	p63 plasma cell antigen, kappa and lambda light chains
Leukaemia	
Common acute lymphoblastic leukaemia (cALL)	CD79a, high proliferation index
T cell acute lymphoblastic leukaemia (T ALL)	CD3, polyclonal, high proliferation index
Acute myeloid leukaemia (AML)	Myeloperoxidase, neutrophil elastase, CD68
Chronic myeloid leukaemia (CML)	Abnormal cells of multiple lineage
Other rare leukaemias	Identify by cell of origin (see section 3 *Focal disease*)

Table 12.5 Antigens identifiable in routine trephine sections by commercially available antibodies.

Antigen	Suggested clone	Pretreatment
CD20	L26	Nil/microwave/pressure cooking
CD79	JCB117	Microwave/pressure cooking
CD3	Polyclonal	Enzyme/microwave/pressure cooking
CD4	NCL-CD4-1F6	Microwave/pressure cooking
CD5	Dk23	Microwave/pressure cooking plus tyramide enhancement
CD8	C8/144B	Microwave/pressure cooking
CD15	C3D-1	Nil/enzyme
CD23	MHM6	Microwave/pressure cooking plus tyramide enhancement
CD30	Ber-H2	Enzyme/microwave/pressure cooking
CD31	JC70A	Enzyme/microwave/pressure cooking
CD34	QBend 10	Microwave/pressure cooking
CD45RO	UCHL1	Microwave/pressure cooking
CD61	Y2/51	Enzyme/pressure cooking
CD68	KP1 or PGM1	Enzyme/microwave/pressure cooking
Cytokeratin	MNF116	Enzyme/pressure cooking
Desmin	D33	Nil
Epithelial membrane antigen	E29	Nil
Factor VIII-related antigen	F8/86	Enzyme
Glycophorin A	JC170	Nil
Glycophorin C	Ret40f	Enzyme
Hairy cell leukaemia	DBA 44	Enzyme/microwave/pressure cooking
Kappa/lambda light chains	Polyclonal	Enzyme/pressure cooking
Ki-67 antigen	Monoclonal or polyclonal	Microwave/pressure cooking
Cyclin D1	DCS22	Microwave/pressure cooking
Leucocyte common antigen	2B11 and PD7/26	Nil
Myoglobin	Polyclonal	Nil
Myeloid/histiocyte antigen	Mac387	Enzyme
Neuroblastoma	NB84	Nil/enzyme/pressure cooking
Myeloperoxidase	Polyclonal	Microwave/pressure cooking
Neutrophil elastase	NP57	Microwave/pressure cooking
Plasma cell p63	VS38	Microwave/pressure cooking
Proliferating cell nuclear antigen	PC10	Nil/microwave/pressure cooking

ation' and represents an internationally agreed system for classifying antigens and their respective monoclonal antibodies. A CD group is a cluster of antibodies recognizing the same antigen. Where there is a series of related genes giving rise to antigenic variants the CD groups have been subdivided, e.g. CD1 a, b, c or CD11 a and b. These groupings are defined at International Workshops on Human Leucocyte Differentiation Antigens. The first of these was held in Paris in 1982, when 15 CD groups were defined. There have to date been six workshops and the number of Clusters has increased to 166. Although this seems a large number it is nothing compared to the thousands of antibodies, each with their own 'laboratory' names, which have been allocated to the clusters. Thus,

referring to the CD number of an antibody rather than the 'pet' name used by the laboratory which produced it (e.g. CD30 rather than Ber H2), allows greater clarity and understanding between users of immunohistochemistry. There are many important antigens with perfectly good names recognized by reliable antibodies which do not have CD numbers. One should not fall into the trap of thinking these are in some way inferior. Table 12.5 is a summary of the antigens and antibodies that we have found helpful in bone marrow diagnosis. Interested parties can discover more about the CD system from the relevant workshop reports or from a number of antibody companies which have information fact sheets available, e.g. R&D Systems or DAKO a/s.

Index